How to stop snoring while sleeping

The ultimate Guide to stop snoring without surgery

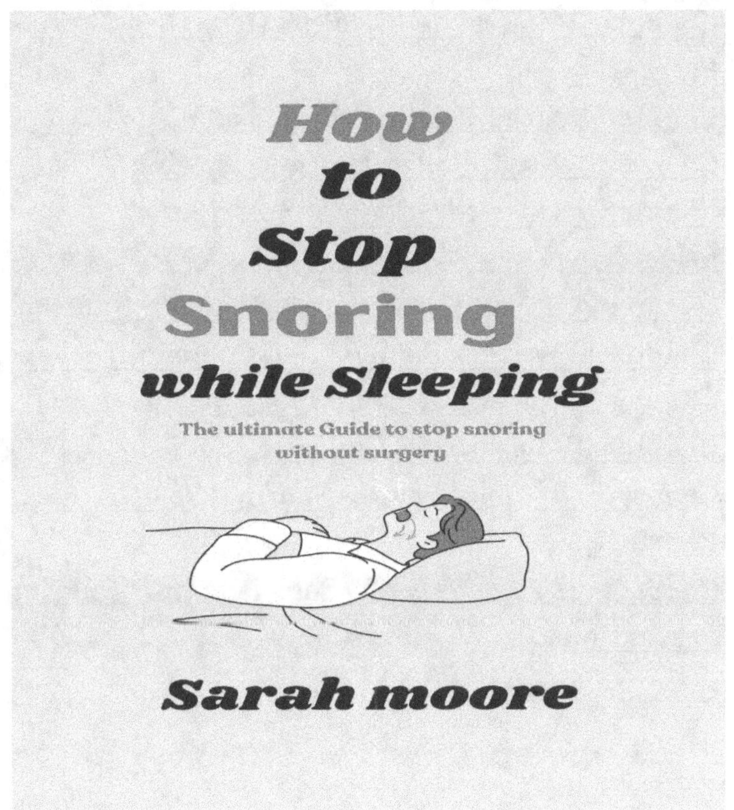

By Sarah Moore

Table of Content

Chapter 1

Introduction to Snoring

Snoring is a common physiological phenomenon that occurs during sleep when the flow of air through the mouth and nose is partially blocked. It results in the production of sound due to the vibration of tissues in the upper airway, primarily the soft palate and uvula. While often considered a minor annoyance, snoring can sometimes indicate underlying health issues or disrupt sleep quality for both the snorer and their sleep partner.

Several factors contribute to snoring:

Anatomy of the Upper Airway: The anatomy of an individual's throat and airway plays a significant role in snoring. People with naturally narrower airways, a low-hanging soft palate, or enlarged tonsils/adenoids are more prone to snoring.

Muscle Tone: Reduced muscle tone in the throat and tongue can cause the airway to narrow during sleep, leading to snoring. This is more common as people age, as muscle tone naturally decreases.

Sleep Position: Sleeping on your back can cause the tongue and soft palate to collapse to the back of the throat, obstructing the airflow and causing snoring.

Obesity: Excess weight, especially around the neck, can put pressure on the airway, making it more likely to collapse during sleep and cause snoring.

Nasal Issues: Conditions like chronic nasal congestion, deviated septum, or allergies can lead to breathing difficulties during sleep, increasing the likelihood of snoring.

Alcohol and Sedatives: The relaxing effect of alcohol and sedatives can cause the muscles in the throat to relax excessively, leading to increased snoring.

Sleep Apnea: Chronic snoring can sometimes be a sign of obstructive sleep apnea (OSA), a condition where breathing repeatedly stops and starts during sleep due to a complete or partial blockage of the upper airway.

Lifestyle Factors: Smoking and exposure to secondhand smoke can irritate and inflame the airway, contributing to snoring. Additionally, poor sleep hygiene, irregular sleep patterns, and sleep deprivation can worsen snoring.

It's important to note that while occasional snoring is usually harmless, chronic and loud snoring might indicate an underlying health issue, like sleep apnea, which can have serious health implications, including cardiovascular problems and daytime sleepiness.

Treatment options for snoring vary based on its underlying causes:

Lifestyle Changes: Losing weight, avoiding alcohol and sedatives close to bedtime, changing sleep positions, and maintaining good sleep hygiene can help alleviate mild snoring.

Nasal Devices: Nasal strips, dilators, and sprays can help open up nasal passages and improve airflow.

Oral Appliances: Dental devices that reposition the jaw and tongue can help prevent the collapse of the airway during sleep.

CPAP Therapy: Continuous Positive Airway Pressure (CPAP) machines are commonly used to treat sleep apnea. They deliver a constant stream of air pressure to keep the airway open.

Surgery: Surgical interventions like Uvulopalatopharyngoplasty (UPPP), genioglossus advancement (GA), or other procedures can be considered for severe cases of snoring or sleep apnea.

If you or someone you know experiences chronic and disruptive snoring, it's advisable to consult a medical professional. A thorough evaluation can help identify the underlying cause and determine the most appropriate treatment approach.

1.1 The Impact of Snoring on Sleep Quality
View other drafts

The impact of snoring on sleep quality is a topic of significant interest in the field of sleep medicine. Snoring is a common occurrence during sleep, often caused by the vibration of relaxed tissues in the throat and nasal passages. While occasional snoring might not have a severe impact, chronic and loud snoring can lead to various negative effects on sleep quality for both the snorer and their bed partner.

For the snorer, frequent snoring can disrupt the natural sleep cycle, preventing them from entering deeper stages of sleep. This disruption can result in fragmented sleep, leading to daytime sleepiness, lack of concentration, and irritability. Snorers may also experience more frequent awakenings during the night, even if they're not fully conscious of them, further impacting the overall sleep architecture.

Additionally, snoring is often associated with a sleep disorder known as obstructive sleep apnea (OSA). OSA occurs when the upper airway becomes partially or completely blocked during sleep, causing breathing to pause or become shallow. These pauses can trigger awakenings throughout the night and lead to a decrease in the overall quality of sleep. OSA is associated with a range of health issues, including cardiovascular problems, high blood pressure, and increased risk of accidents due to daytime sleepiness.

The impact of snoring isn't limited to the snorer alone; it can also affect their bed partner. The noise generated by snoring can lead to disturbances in the partner's sleep, causing them to experience sleep fragmentation, difficulty falling back asleep, and reduced sleep quality.

Over time, these disruptions can strain the partner's well-being and potentially lead to conflicts or separate sleep arrangements.

Addressing the impact of snoring on sleep quality involves both lifestyle modifications and medical interventions. For mild cases, individuals might be advised to make changes such as sleeping on their side, maintaining a healthy weight, avoiding alcohol before bedtime, and using nasal strips to improve airflow. In more severe cases, medical interventions like continuous positive airway pressure (CPAP) therapy might be recommended to treat sleep apnea and alleviate snoring.

In conclusion, snoring can have a significant impact on sleep quality for both the snorer and their bed partner. Its potential to disrupt the sleep cycle and contribute to sleep disorders like sleep apnea underscores the importance of addressing this issue to ensure overall well-being and restful sleep.

1.2 Understanding the Causes of Snoring

Snoring is a common phenomenon that occurs during sleep, characterized by the vibration of the tissues in the throat and nasal passages. It can be caused by various factors, both anatomical and lifestyle-related. Here's an in-depth look at some of the key causes of snoring:

Anatomical Factors:

Nasal Congestion: When the nasal passages are partially blocked due to allergies, colds, or sinus infections, airflow can be restricted, leading to snoring.
Deviated Septum: A deviated nasal septum can cause uneven airflow through the nostrils, contributing to snoring.
Enlarged Tonsils or Adenoids: In children and adults, enlarged tonsils or adenoids can obstruct the airway and trigger snoring.

Soft Palate and Uvula: An elongated or relaxed soft palate and uvula can obstruct the airway and cause snoring.

Obesity: Excess fat tissue around the neck and throat can put pressure on the airway, narrowing it and causing snoring.

Lifestyle Factors:

Sleep Position: Sleeping on your back can cause the tongue and soft palate to collapse to the back of the throat, obstructing airflow and resulting in snoring.

Alcohol and Sedatives: Consuming alcohol or certain sedatives relaxes the muscles in the throat, increasing the likelihood of snoring.

Smoking: Smoking irritates and inflames the tissues in the throat, contributing to snoring.

Obesity: Apart from its anatomical impact, obesity can also lead to poor muscle tone in the throat, increasing the likelihood of snoring.

Sleep Deprivation: Not getting enough sleep can lead to increased relaxation of throat muscles, leading to snoring.

Sleep Apnea: A more serious condition, sleep apnea involves repeated pauses in breathing

during sleep due to a collapse of the airway. Snoring is a common symptom of sleep apnea.
Age and Gender:

Age: As people age, the throat muscles naturally lose some tone, increasing the risk of snoring.
Gender: Men are more likely to snore compared to women, possibly due to differences in throat anatomy.
Medical Conditions:

Hypothyroidism: An underactive thyroid can lead to weight gain and throat muscle relaxation, contributing to snoring.
Acromegaly: This hormonal disorder causes the enlargement of certain body parts, including the tongue and soft palate, which can lead to snoring.
Understanding the causes of snoring is crucial for finding appropriate solutions. Lifestyle changes such as maintaining a healthy weight, sleeping on your side, avoiding alcohol before bedtime, and addressing allergies can help alleviate snoring. In cases of persistent or severe snoring, it's advisable to consult a medical

professional for proper diagnosis and treatment options.

1.3 The Importance of Addressing Snoring

Snoring is a common phenomenon that occurs when airflow is partially obstructed during sleep, causing the tissues in the throat to vibrate and create sound. While it might be seen as a mere nuisance, snoring can actually have more profound implications, warranting attention and intervention.

Health Implications: Snoring can disrupt the quality of sleep for both the snorer and their bed partner. This disrupted sleep can lead to daytime fatigue, difficulty concentrating, and irritability. Moreover, chronic snoring might be an indicator of a more serious condition known as obstructive sleep apnea (OSA), where the airway repeatedly collapses during sleep, causing oxygen levels to drop. OSA is linked to a higher risk of cardiovascular problems, including hypertension, heart disease, and stroke.

Relationship Strain: Snoring can strain relationships due to the disturbance it causes to the partner's sleep. Sleep disruptions can lead to resentment and communication breakdowns, impacting the overall quality of the relationship. Addressing snoring can not only improve the snorer's health but also nurture healthier relationships.

Quality of Life: The lack of restful sleep due to snoring can have a negative impact on overall quality of life. Daytime drowsiness can affect job performance, concentration, and the ability to enjoy daily activities. Addressing snoring can lead to improved sleep quality, resulting in enhanced energy levels, mood, and overall well-being.

Safety Concerns: Severe snoring coupled with sleep apnea can increase the risk of accidents, especially while engaging in activities that require alertness, such as driving. The impaired cognitive function resulting from sleep disruptions can compromise reaction times and decision-making abilities.

Medical Costs: Untreated snoring and sleep apnea can lead to more serious health issues, resulting in increased medical costs over time. By addressing snoring and its potential underlying causes, individuals can mitigate the risk of developing chronic health conditions that require more extensive medical treatment.

Treatment Options: The importance of addressing snoring is underscored by the availability of various treatment options. Lifestyle changes, such as weight loss, avoiding alcohol and sedatives, and sleeping on one's side, can help alleviate snoring. Medical devices like CPAP (Continuous Positive Airway Pressure) machines are effective for managing sleep apnea. In some cases, surgical interventions might be necessary to correct anatomical issues that contribute to snoring.

In conclusion, snoring should not be dismissed as a minor inconvenience. Its potential health implications, impact on relationships, and overall well-being highlight the need for timely intervention. By addressing snoring through lifestyle changes, medical treatments, and seeking professional guidance, individuals can enjoy better sleep, improved health, and a higher quality of life.

Chapter 2

The Science Behind Snoring

Snoring is a common phenomenon that occurs during sleep and is caused by the vibration of tissues in the airway. The science behind snoring involves several factors, including anatomy, airflow dynamics, and muscle tone.

Anatomy of the Airway: The airway consists of various structures, including the nasal passages, throat (pharynx), and the base of the tongue. When we sleep, the muscles that keep these structures open relax. This relaxation can lead to partial blockage or narrowing of the airway.

Airflow Dynamics: As we breathe during sleep, air moves through the narrowed or partially blocked airway. The soft tissues in the airway, such as the uvula and the soft palate, can vibrate as the air passes over them. These vibrations produce the sound we know as snoring. The narrower the airway, the greater the turbulence of airflow, and the louder the snoring tends to be.

Muscle Tone: The muscles that help keep the airway open can lose tone during sleep, especially in deeper stages of sleep. This relaxation can exacerbate the narrowing of the airway, leading to more pronounced snoring. Factors like alcohol consumption, sedative medications, and sleeping on one's back can further relax these muscles.

Risk Factors: Certain factors increase the likelihood of snoring. These include obesity, as excess fat around the neck can put pressure on the airway; age, as muscle tone naturally decreases with age; nasal congestion, which can obstruct airflow; and anatomical variations, such as having a deviated septum or large tonsils.

Sleep Apnea Connection: Snoring can also be associated with a more serious condition called sleep apnea. Sleep apnea occurs when the airway is completely blocked for brief periods, leading to interrupted breathing and repeated awakenings during sleep. Loud, chronic snoring is often a key symptom of sleep apnea.

Treatment Options: Treatment for snoring depends on its underlying cause. Lifestyle changes such as weight loss, sleeping on one's side, and avoiding alcohol before bedtime can help reduce snoring. In cases of sleep apnea, continuous positive airway pressure (CPAP) therapy may be recommended. This involves wearing a mask that delivers a continuous flow of air to keep the airway open.

Surgical Interventions: For severe cases of snoring or sleep apnea, surgical interventions might be considered. These can include procedures to remove excess tissue from the throat, correct anatomical abnormalities, or stiffen the soft palate to reduce vibrations.

In summary, snoring is a complex phenomenon involving the interaction of various anatomical and physiological factors. Understanding the science behind snoring can help individuals and healthcare professionals identify the underlying causes and determine the most appropriate treatment options. If you or someone you know is experiencing persistent and disruptive snoring, it's advisable to consult a medical professional for a proper evaluation and guidance.

2.1 Anatomy of the Respiratory System

The respiratory system is a complex anatomical structure responsible for the exchange of gases between the body and the environment. It consists of various organs and structures that work together to facilitate the intake of oxygen and the removal of carbon dioxide. Here's an in-depth overview of the anatomy of the respiratory system:

Nasal Cavity and Mouth:
The process of respiration begins with the inhalation of air through either the nasal cavity

or the mouth. The nasal cavity is lined with mucous membranes and tiny hair-like structures called cilia that help filter, warm, and humidify the incoming air.

Pharynx:
The air then passes through the pharynx, which is a common pathway for both air and food. The epiglottis, a flap of tissue, prevents food from entering the trachea during swallowing.

Larynx:
The air then enters the larynx, commonly known as the voice box, where sound is produced. The vocal cords within the larynx can be adjusted to produce different pitches and tones.

Trachea:
From the larynx, the air moves into the trachea, a tube reinforced with cartilage rings that prevents its collapse during inhalation. The trachea branches into two smaller tubes known as the bronchi—one leading to each lung.

Bronchial Tree:

Within the lungs, the bronchi continue to divide into smaller and narrower tubes called bronchioles. These bronchioles eventually lead to clusters of air sacs called alveoli.

Alveoli:

Alveoli are the primary sites of gas exchange in the respiratory system. These tiny sacs are surrounded by capillaries, allowing for the exchange of oxygen from the air into the bloodstream and the removal of carbon dioxide from the blood into the air.

Lungs:

The lungs are the major organs of the respiratory system and are divided into lobes. The right lung has three lobes, while the left lung has two due to the space occupied by the heart. The lungs are surrounded by a double-layered membrane called the pleura, which helps facilitate breathing movements.

Diaphragm:

The diaphragm is a dome-shaped muscle that plays a crucial role in respiration. When it contracts, it flattens, increasing the volume of the thoracic cavity and causing inhalation. Relaxation of the diaphragm leads to exhalation.

The respiratory system's primary function is to supply the body with oxygen while eliminating carbon dioxide, a waste product of metabolism. The intricate network of structures within the respiratory system ensures that this exchange occurs efficiently, enabling the body's cells to function properly.

Keep in mind that this is a simplified overview, and there are many additional details and nuances within the respiratory system's anatomy that contribute to its functionality.

2.2 How Snoring Occurs

Snoring occurs due to the vibration of tissues in the throat and nasal passages during sleep. When you sleep, the muscles in your throat and tongue relax, causing the airway to narrow. As you breathe, the flow of air causes these relaxed tissues to vibrate, producing the sound of snoring. Factors such as obesity, nasal congestion, alcohol consumption, sleep position, and anatomical features like a deviated septum can contribute to snoring. In more severe cases, snoring might be linked to sleep apnea, a condition where breathing repeatedly stops and starts during sleep due to a complete or partial obstruction of the airway.

2.3 Different Types of Snoring

Snoring is a common sleep-related phenomenon that occurs when the flow of air through the mouth and nose is partially blocked during sleep, causing the surrounding tissues to vibrate and create noise. There are various types of snoring, each with distinct underlying causes. Here are some in-depth explanations of different types of snoring:

Nasal Snoring: Nasal congestion, allergies, or structural issues such as a deviated septum can lead to nasal snoring. When the nasal passages are obstructed, the airflow becomes turbulent, resulting in snoring sounds.

Mouth Breathers Snoring: Some individuals tend to breathe through their mouths while sleeping. This can cause the tissues in the throat and mouth to become loose, leading to snoring. This type of snoring can often be reduced by encouraging nasal breathing.

Tongue-based Snoring: The tongue falling backward during sleep can partially block the airway, causing snoring. This type of snoring is more common in individuals who sleep on their back. Tongue-retaining devices or positional therapy can help address this type of snoring.

Palatal Flutter Snoring: This occurs when the tissues in the roof of the mouth (soft palate and uvula) vibrate due to turbulent airflow. It's often associated with the relaxation of these tissues during sleep and can be influenced by factors like alcohol consumption and sleep position.

Uvula Vibrations: The uvula, a fleshy tissue hanging at the back of the throat, can vibrate and cause snoring when airflow passes over it. Sometimes, snoring caused by the uvula can lead to sleep apnea, a more serious condition where breathing is briefly interrupted during sleep.

Obstructive Sleep Apnea (OSA) Snoring: While not all snoring is indicative of sleep apnea, loud and chronic snoring could be a sign of OSA. OSA occurs when the airway is repeatedly partially or completely blocked during sleep, leading to interrupted breathing and oxygen deprivation. It's a serious condition that requires medical attention.

Positional Snoring: Sleep position can influence snoring. People who sleep on their backs are more likely to snore, as gravity causes the relaxed tissues in the throat to collapse into the airway. Positional therapy involves encouraging sleeping on one's side to reduce snoring.

Lifestyle-related Snoring: Lifestyle factors such as obesity, alcohol consumption, smoking, and certain medications can contribute to snoring. Excess weight, for example, can lead to increased fatty tissue in the throat, narrowing the airway and promoting snoring.

Primary Snoring: Some individuals snore without having any underlying medical condition or sleep disorder. This is referred to as primary snoring and is typically less severe than snoring associated with sleep apnea.

It's important to note that snoring can have various causes and contributing factors. If snoring is affecting your sleep quality or that of your partner, it's advisable to consult a medical professional or a sleep specialist. They can help identify the specific type of snoring and recommend appropriate treatments or interventions to address the issue.

Chapter 3

Lifestyle Modifications for Snoring Prevention

In-depth explanation of lifestyle modifications that can help prevent snoring.

Maintain a Healthy Weight: Carrying excess weight, especially around the neck area, can lead to narrowing of the airway, which increases the likelihood of snoring. Engaging in regular exercise and following a balanced diet can help you maintain a healthy weight and reduce snoring.

Sleep Position: Sleeping on your back can cause the tongue and soft palate to collapse to the back of the throat, obstructing the airway and causing snoring. Sleeping on your side can alleviate this issue and reduce snoring. You can use pillows or devices to encourage sleeping on your side.

Avoid Alcohol and Sedatives: Alcohol and sedatives relax the muscles in your throat, which can lead to increased snoring. Avoiding or minimizing the consumption of these substances, especially close to bedtime, can help reduce snoring.

Stay Hydrated: Dehydration can make the secretions in your nose and soft palate stickier, leading to snoring. Drinking plenty of water throughout the day can help keep these areas lubricated.

Nasal Congestion Management: If you have nasal congestion due to allergies or other factors, it can lead to breathing through your mouth and increase the chances of snoring. Using saline nasal sprays, allergy medications, or a humidifier in your bedroom can help alleviate congestion.

Elevate Your Head: Using an extra pillow or elevating the head of your bed by a few inches can help keep your airways more open, reducing the likelihood of snoring.

Practice Good Sleep Hygiene: Establishing a regular sleep schedule and ensuring you get adequate sleep can help prevent snoring. Fatigue can lead to increased relaxation of throat muscles, contributing to snoring.

Treat Sleep Apnea: If your snoring is accompanied by pauses in breathing or choking sounds, it could be a sign of sleep apnea. Consult a medical professional for proper diagnosis and treatment options.

Avoid Large Meals Before Bed: Eating large meals or heavy, rich foods shortly before bedtime can put pressure on your diaphragm and increase the likelihood of snoring. Try to finish meals at least a few hours before sleeping.

Quit Smoking: Smoking irritates the tissues in your throat and can cause inflammation, leading to snoring. Quitting smoking not only benefits your overall health but can also reduce snoring.

Remember that individual responses to lifestyle changes vary, and it might take time to see significant improvements. If snoring persists despite trying these modifications, or if it's causing sleep disturbances for you or your partner, it's a good idea to consult a healthcare professional for a proper evaluation and guidance.

3.1 Maintaining a Healthy Weight to help cope with snoring

Maintaining a healthy weight can indeed play a significant role in managing and reducing snoring. Snoring occurs when there is an obstruction or partial blockage in the airway during sleep, causing vibrations in the tissues of the throat. Excess weight, especially around the neck area, can contribute to this obstruction and lead to snoring. Here's an in-depth look at how maintaining a healthy weight can help cope with snoring:

Reduced Fat Accumulation: Carrying excess body weight, particularly around the neck, can result in the accumulation of fatty tissues in the throat and neck area. This can narrow the airway, making it more likely for snoring to occur as air struggles to pass through the narrowed space.

Decreased Pressure on Airways: A higher body mass index (BMI) can increase the pressure on the airways, leading to their collapse or narrowing during sleep. Losing weight can alleviate this pressure and allow the airways to remain open, reducing the chances of snoring.

Improved Muscle Tone: Losing weight through a combination of healthy eating and regular exercise can help improve muscle tone in the throat and neck area. Stronger muscles are less likely to collapse or vibrate during sleep, which can help prevent snoring.

Less Inflammation: Obesity is associated with inflammation in the body, including in the tissues of the throat. Inflamed tissues are more likely to obstruct the airway and contribute to snoring. By maintaining a healthy weight, you can help reduce inflammation and improve the overall health of your airways.

Sleep Apnea Management: Sleep apnea is a more severe condition often linked to snoring. It involves pauses in breathing during sleep due to airway obstruction. Excess weight is a significant risk factor for sleep apnea. Losing weight can reduce the severity of sleep apnea and consequently decrease snoring.

Lifestyle Changes: Achieving and maintaining a healthy weight involves adopting a healthier lifestyle. This can include making dietary changes, engaging in regular physical activity, and managing stress. These changes can collectively contribute to better sleep quality and reduced snoring.

Consultation with Professionals: If snoring persists even after weight loss efforts, it's essential to consult with healthcare professionals. They can evaluate your condition, recommend further interventions if necessary, and provide guidance on managing snoring and its underlying causes.

In conclusion, maintaining a healthy weight is an important aspect of managing snoring. It addresses multiple factors that contribute to snoring, such as airway obstruction, inflammation, and muscle tone. However, individual responses may vary, and it's always best to seek guidance from healthcare professionals for a comprehensive approach to snoring management.

3.2 Dietary Changes to Reduce Snoring

Snoring is often influenced by various factors, including diet. Making specific dietary changes can potentially help reduce snoring by addressing underlying causes. Here are some in-depth dietary changes that could be considered to alleviate snoring:

Maintain a Healthy Weight: Carrying excess weight, especially around the neck, can put pressure on the airways and lead to snoring. Adopting a balanced diet and engaging in regular physical activity can help with weight management.

Reduce Inflammatory Foods: Inflammation in the throat and nasal passages can contribute to snoring. Cutting down on highly processed foods, sugary snacks, and foods high in trans fats may help reduce inflammation.

Limit Alcohol Intake: Alcohol relaxes the muscles in the throat, which can obstruct the airway and increase the likelihood of snoring. Moderating or avoiding alcohol consumption, especially before bedtime, can help minimize this effect.

Avoid Heavy Meals Before Bed: Eating large meals close to bedtime can put pressure on the stomach, causing it to push against the diaphragm and affect breathing. Aim to have dinner at least a few hours before going to sleep.

Hydrate Properly: Dehydration can lead to stickiness in the throat and nasal passages, potentially increasing the vibrations that cause snoring. Stay hydrated throughout the day to prevent this.

Consider Anti-Inflammatory Foods: Incorporating foods rich in antioxidants and anti-inflammatory compounds, such as fruits, vegetables, whole grains, and healthy fats (like those found in nuts and olive oil), can help reduce inflammation in the airways.

Spice It Up: Spices like turmeric, ginger, and garlic have anti-inflammatory properties and may help improve airflow. Including them in your meals could be beneficial.

Include Omega-3 Fatty Acids: Foods like fatty fish (salmon, mackerel, sardines) and flaxseeds contain omega-3 fatty acids, which have anti-inflammatory effects and might contribute to improved breathing.

Avoid Dairy Before Bed: Some people are sensitive to dairy products, which can lead to excess mucus production and congestion. If dairy seems to exacerbate your snoring, consider avoiding it before sleep.

Elevate the Head: While not directly related to diet, using an extra pillow or adjusting your sleeping position can help keep the airways open and reduce the chances of snoring.

Remember that individual responses to dietary changes vary, so it's essential to monitor how your body responds and consult with a healthcare professional before making significant modifications to your diet. Addressing snoring comprehensively may involve a combination of lifestyle changes, including dietary adjustments, regular exercise, and good sleep hygiene.

3.3 Limiting Alcohol and Smoking to prevent snoring

In-depth explanation on how limiting alcohol and smoking can help prevent snoring.

Alcohol:
Alcohol acts as a depressant on the central nervous system, causing relaxation of the muscles in the body, including the muscles in the throat. When these muscles relax excessively, the airway can become narrower, and the tissues in the throat may vibrate more when air passes through during breathing, leading to snoring. Additionally, alcohol consumption can also lead to an increase in inflammation and fluid retention in the throat, further contributing to airway obstruction and snoring.

Smoking:
Smoking damages the respiratory system in various ways. It irritates and inflames the tissues of the throat and the airway, leading to a swelling of the tissues. This inflammation and swelling can narrow the air passage, making it more likely

for snoring to occur. Smoking also causes a build-up of mucus in the airway, which can obstruct airflow and contribute to snoring. Moreover, smoking has been linked to an increased risk of sleep apnea, a condition characterized by repeated interruptions in breathing during sleep, which is closely related to snoring.

Why Limiting Alcohol and Smoking Helps:
By limiting alcohol consumption and quitting smoking, you can take important steps to reduce the likelihood of snoring and improve your overall sleep quality. Avoiding alcohol before bedtime helps to keep the muscles of the throat from becoming overly relaxed, preventing them from obstructing the airway. Similarly, quitting smoking reduces inflammation and swelling in the throat tissues, allowing for improved airflow during sleep. Overall, these lifestyle changes not only help prevent snoring but also have a positive impact on your respiratory and cardiovascular health.

Additional Tips to Prevent Snoring:

Maintain a healthy weight: Excess weight, especially around the neck, can put pressure on the airway and contribute to snoring.

Sleep on your side: Sleeping on your back can cause your tongue and soft palate to collapse to the back of your throat, obstructing airflow. Sleeping on your side can help keep the airway open.

Stay hydrated: Drinking plenty of water helps to keep the tissues in the throat from becoming sticky and causing vibration.

Elevate your head: Using a slightly elevated pillow or adjusting the angle of your bed can help keep the airway open.

Remember that individual responses to these lifestyle changes may vary. If snoring persists despite making these changes, or if you suspect you have sleep apnea, it's important to consult a healthcare professional for a proper diagnosis and personalized treatment plan.

3.4 Regular Exercise and its Effects on Snoring

Regular exercise can have a notable impact on snoring, a common sleep-related issue. Engaging in consistent physical activity can contribute to several factors that help alleviate or even reduce snoring.

Weight Management: One of the primary ways exercise helps with snoring is by aiding in weight management. Excess weight, especially around the neck area, can lead to the narrowing of the airway during sleep, which in turn increases the likelihood of snoring. Regular exercise helps burn calories, reduce body fat, and maintain a healthy weight, which can mitigate this issue.

Muscle Tone: Exercise promotes muscle tone and strength throughout the body, including the muscles of the throat and tongue. Strengthening these muscles can help prevent them from collapsing and obstructing the airway during sleep, thereby reducing snoring.

Improved Sleep Quality: Regular physical activity has been linked to improved sleep quality. Getting sufficient, restful sleep is crucial for reducing snoring, as fatigue and poor sleep can exacerbate the relaxation of throat muscles, contributing to snoring.

Reduced Nasal Congestion: Certain exercises can help improve nasal airflow and reduce congestion. This is particularly important because nasal congestion can lead to mouth breathing, which often intensifies snoring.

Stress Reduction: Exercise is known to reduce stress and anxiety levels. Lower stress levels can promote more relaxed sleep, which can in turn reduce the likelihood of snoring.

Lifestyle Changes: Engaging in regular exercise often goes hand-in-hand with adopting a healthier lifestyle. This might include dietary improvements and the avoidance of habits that worsen snoring, such as alcohol consumption and smoking.

Consistency Matters: While exercise can have positive effects on snoring, it's important to note that results may take time. Consistency is key; the benefits are more likely to be noticeable with regular, ongoing physical activity.

It's important to consult with a medical professional before starting any new exercise regimen, especially if you have underlying health conditions. Additionally, while exercise can help with snoring, it might not completely eliminate the issue for everyone. If snoring persists despite lifestyle changes, it's advisable to seek medical advice to rule out any underlying sleep disorders or health concerns.

Remember, individual experiences may vary, and a multifaceted approach that includes exercise, dietary adjustments, and healthy sleep habits can be the most effective way to address snoring.

Chapter 4

Sleep Positions and Snoring

Snoring is often influenced by various factors, including sleep position. The way you position your body during sleep can impact the airflow in your throat, which in turn can affect snoring. Here's an exploration of different sleep positions and their potential effects on snoring:

Back Sleeping (Supine Position): Sleeping on your back can lead to the base of your tongue and soft palate collapsing to the back wall of your throat, narrowing the airway. This restricted airflow can result in vibration of the tissues, causing the sound of snoring. Back sleeping is often associated with increased snoring and even sleep apnea.

Side Sleeping (Lateral Position): Sleeping on your side, particularly on your left side, is generally considered one of the best positions for reducing snoring. This position helps keep the airway open and reduces the likelihood of the tongue and soft palate obstructing the airflow.

Stomach Sleeping (Prone Position): While less common, sleeping on your stomach can also impact snoring. This position can sometimes cause strain on the neck and may not be as effective at keeping the airway open. However, some people find relief from snoring in this position, especially if they naturally breathe through their nose.

Elevated Head Position: Using a thicker pillow or elevating the head of the bed can also help reduce snoring for some people. This elevation can help keep the airway more open and decrease the likelihood of tissue vibrations.

Combination Position: Many people naturally shift between different positions during the night. If you tend to snore more when on your back, try using pillows or positioning aids to encourage side sleeping.

It's important to note that individual factors play a significant role in how sleep position affects snoring. Factors such as weight, body structure, nasal congestion, and sleep disorders can all influence snoring patterns. For instance, someone with nasal congestion might snore less when sleeping on their side to avoid obstructing their already-congested airway.

If snoring is a persistent issue, it's advisable to consult a medical professional. They can help identify the underlying causes of snoring and provide recommendations tailored to your specific situation. Lifestyle changes, positional therapy devices, or medical interventions may be suggested to address snoring and improve overall sleep quality.

Remember that while sleep position can play a role, it's just one factor among many that contribute to snoring. Addressing other potential factors, such as obesity, allergies, alcohol consumption, and smoking, can also have a positive impact on reducing snoring.

4.1 The Impact of Sleep Position on Snoring

Snoring is a common sleep-related phenomenon caused by the vibration of tissues in the upper airway during breathing. The position in which a person sleeps can have a significant influence on the occurrence and intensity of snoring. Different sleep positions can affect the airway's anatomy and muscle tone, leading to variations in airflow and tissue vibration, which ultimately contribute to snoring.

Here's a breakdown of how various sleep positions can impact snoring:

Supine (Back) Position: Sleeping on your back can often lead to increased snoring. This position tends to relax the muscles of the throat and tongue, causing the airway to narrow. As a result, airflow becomes turbulent, and the tissues are more likely to vibrate, producing the sound of snoring.

Side Position: Sleeping on your side is generally considered the best position to reduce snoring. This position helps keep the airway open and prevents the tongue and soft palate from collapsing backward. Side sleeping can decrease the likelihood of tissue vibration and turbulent airflow, leading to less snoring.

Prone (Stomach) Position: While less common, sleeping on your stomach can also influence snoring. This position might help keep the airway more open compared to the supine position. However, for some individuals, it could cause strain on the neck and back and may not be the most comfortable option.

Head Elevation: Elevating the head and upper body during sleep can be effective in reducing snoring. This position helps counteract the effects of gravity on the throat muscles and can prevent airway collapse.

Combination of Positions: Some individuals naturally change positions throughout the night. For example, someone might start on their side but end up on their back. Positional therapy involves using various methods to encourage sleeping in a specific position to reduce snoring.

It's important to note that while sleep position plays a significant role in snoring, it's not the sole factor. Other factors such as obesity, alcohol consumption, sleep apnea, nasal congestion, and anatomical features also contribute to snoring.

If snoring is a persistent issue, it's advisable to consult a healthcare professional. They can evaluate whether sleep position is the primary cause of snoring or if there are other underlying factors that need to be addressed. Lifestyle changes, positional therapy devices, and, in some cases, medical interventions might be recommended to alleviate snoring and improve sleep quality.

4.2 Tips for Encouraging Side Sleeping

Here are some in-depth tips for encouraging side sleeping:

Mattress and Pillow Selection:
Choose a mattress and pillows that provide adequate support and comfort for side sleeping. A mattress that is medium-firm can help maintain proper spinal alignment, while pillows that are higher under the neck and lower under the head provide good neck support.

Body Pillow Usage:
Placing a body pillow between your knees and arms can help maintain a neutral spinal alignment while preventing your top leg from pulling your spine out of alignment.

Sleeping Environment:
Create a sleep-conducive environment by keeping your room dark, quiet, and at a comfortable temperature. This can encourage deeper sleep and make side sleeping more comfortable.

Positional Training:
If you're not used to sleeping, practice during daytime naps. Gradually, your body will become accustomed to the position, making it more natural during the night.

Bedtime Routine:
Develop a calming bedtime routine to signal your body that it's time to wind down. Activities like reading, gentle stretching, or meditation can help relax your mind and body, making sleeping more comfortable.

Adjustment Period:
Understand that switching sleep positions might take some time. Be patient with yourself as your body adjusts to the new sleeping posture.

Pillow Support:
Proper pillow placement is crucial. Your head should be aligned with your spine, not too high or too low. Consider using a contoured pillow that cradles your head and neck in the side sleeping position.

Pain Management:
If you experience discomfort, particularly in your shoulder or hip, consider using extra pillows for support. Placing a pillow under your waist can help align your spine and alleviate pressure points.

Avoiding Stomach Sleeping:
Sleeping on your stomach can strain your neck and spine. Try to gradually transition from stomach sleeping to side sleeping to reduce the risk of discomfort and pain.

Consistency:
Once you've adapted to side sleeping, try to maintain this position consistently. Consistency in sleep posture can contribute to better overall sleep quality.

Remember, it's important to find the sleep position that feels most comfortable and suits your body's needs. If you have specific medical concerns or chronic pain, it's advisable to consult a healthcare professional for personalized guidance.

4.3 Specially Designed Pillows and Devices for Sleep Positioning

Specially designed pillows and devices for sleep positioning have gained popularity as people become more aware of the importance of quality sleep. These products aim to enhance sleep comfort and address specific issues such as snoring, sleep apnea, acid reflux, and musculoskeletal pain.

One common type of specially designed pillow is the cervical pillow, which is contoured to support the natural curve of the neck and promote proper spinal alignment. This can alleviate neck pain and reduce the risk of waking up with stiffness. Additionally, wedge pillows are often used to elevate the upper body, helping to alleviate symptoms of acid reflux, congestion, and breathing difficulties during sleep.

For individuals with sleep apnea, specialized pillows and devices like positional therapy aids are available. These products encourage side-sleeping, which is known to be beneficial for reducing the severity of sleep apnea symptoms. Positional therapy devices can include various forms, such as inflatable cushions or wearable belts, which help discourage back sleeping.

Pregnancy pillows are another category designed to support pregnant women during sleep. These pillows are shaped to provide comfort and support for the changing body contours during pregnancy, helping to alleviate back pain and discomfort.

Snoring is another common sleep issue that can be addressed through specially designed pillows. Anti-snoring pillows often incorporate features like raised edges to encourage side-sleeping and prevent the airway from becoming obstructed. Some products even have built-in sensors that can detect snoring and gently adjust the pillow's shape to encourage a change in sleeping position.

It's important to note that while these pillows and devices can offer benefits for certain sleep-related concerns, individual experiences may vary. Consulting with a healthcare professional before investing in such products is advisable, especially if you have underlying medical conditions. Additionally, combining these products with good sleep hygiene practices, such as maintaining a consistent sleep schedule and creating a conducive sleep environment, can contribute to overall sleep improvement.

Chapter 5

Nasal Congestion and Snoring

Nasal congestion is the result of swollen nasal passages, usually due to inflammation caused by factors like allergies, colds, or sinus infections. This can obstruct the flow of air, making breathing through the nose difficult. When you're congested, the body often switches to breathing through the mouth, which can lead to snoring.

Snoring occurs when the flow of air through the mouth and nose is partially blocked during sleep. This obstruction causes the surrounding tissues (like the uvula and soft palate) to vibrate, resulting in the characteristic snoring sound. Nasal congestion contributes to snoring by narrowing the nasal passages, forcing more air to pass through the mouth, and increasing the likelihood of tissue vibration.

There are several interconnected factors that can lead to both nasal congestion and snoring:

Anatomy: Some people have naturally narrower airways or structures that are more prone to vibration, which can contribute to both conditions.

Allergies: Allergic reactions can cause inflammation in the nasal passages, leading to congestion. This can occur due to sensitivities to pollen, pet dander, dust mites, and more.

Infections: Colds, flu, and sinus infections can result in swollen nasal passages and congestion.

Deviated Septum: A deviated septum, where the wall separating the nostrils is crooked, can obstruct airflow and contribute to congestion and snoring.

Obesity: Excess weight, especially around the neck, can put pressure on the airways and lead to snoring. It can also contribute to inflammation and congestion.

Sleep Position: Sleeping on your back can cause the tongue and soft palate to collapse to the back of the throat, potentially causing snoring. Nasal congestion can exacerbate this by forcing mouth breathing.

Alcohol and Sedatives: These substances relax the muscles in the throat, increasing the likelihood of airway obstruction and snoring.

Addressing nasal congestion and snoring often involves identifying and managing the underlying causes:

Nasal Sprays: Over-the-counter or prescription nasal sprays can help reduce congestion by shrinking swollen blood vessels in the nasal passages.

Allergy Management: If allergies are the cause, allergen avoidance and medications like antihistamines can help manage congestion.

Hydration and Humidification: Staying hydrated and using a humidifier in your bedroom can keep nasal passages moist and reduce congestion.

Positional Changes: Sleeping on your side instead of your back can reduce the likelihood of snoring, as can elevating your head slightly.

Weight Management: If excess weight is contributing to your snoring, losing weight can help alleviate the issue.

Medical Interventions: In cases of severe snoring and congestion, medical interventions like surgery to correct a deviated septum or remove excess tissue might be considered.

Remember that persistent snoring and congestion can sometimes be indicative of a more serious condition called sleep apnea, where breathing is repeatedly interrupted during sleep.

If you're concerned, it's best to consult a healthcare professional for an accurate diagnosis and appropriate treatment recommendations.

5.1 Understanding Nasal Congestion and its Relationship to Snoring

Nasal congestion is a common condition where the tissues lining the nasal passages become swollen and inflamed, leading to a blocked or stuffy nose. It can result from various factors such as allergies, infections, or irritants. Nasal congestion can significantly impact one's breathing, sleep quality, and even contribute to snoring.

When the nasal passages are congested, airflow through the nose becomes restricted. This forces individuals to rely more on breathing through their mouth, especially during sleep. Breathing through the mouth can create turbulence in the airway, leading to the vibration of soft tissues in the throat, which is a common cause of snoring.

The relationship between nasal congestion and snoring is a two-fold process. First, nasal congestion can make it harder for individuals to breathe through their nose while asleep. This leads to increased efforts to breathe, causing negative pressure in the airway, which in turn contributes to the collapse of soft tissues like the uvula, palate, and tongue. This obstruction causes the characteristic sound of snoring.

Second, nasal congestion often leads to an increase in inflammation and mucus production in the upper airway. This excess mucus and inflammation can further narrow the airway, making it even more likely for the soft tissues to vibrate and cause snoring sounds.

Addressing nasal congestion can be an effective way to reduce snoring. Treating the underlying cause of congestion, such as allergies or infections, can alleviate the issue. Over-the-counter or prescription nasal decongestants can help reduce inflammation and open up the nasal passages. Nasal strips can also be used to physically widen the nostrils and improve airflow. In some cases, a medical professional might recommend surgical procedures to correct structural issues in the nasal passages, which can also alleviate snoring.

In conclusion, understanding the relationship between nasal congestion and snoring is crucial in managing sleep-related breathing issues. Addressing nasal congestion through various methods can not only improve sleep quality but also contribute to reducing snoring and its associated complications.

5.2 Remedies for Clearing Nasal Passages

Here are some in-depth remedies for clearing nasal passages:

Saline Nasal Irrigation: Saline solution (a mixture of salt and water) is used to rinse the nasal passages. This helps to thin mucus and clear out irritants, allergens, and bacteria. You can use a neti pot or a squeeze bottle to gently flush the saline solution through one nostril and let it drain out of the other.

Steam Inhalation: Inhaling steam can help loosen mucus and provide relief from congestion. Boil water, pour it into a bowl, and lean over the bowl with a towel over your head. Breathe in the steam for about 10 minutes.

Nasal Decongestant Sprays: Over-the-counter nasal sprays containing decongestants like oxymetazoline can provide quick relief by constricting blood vessels in the nasal passages. However, these should be used for a maximum of three days to avoid rebound congestion.

Humidifiers: Using a humidifier in your room adds moisture to the air, preventing the nasal passages from drying out and becoming congested. This is especially helpful during dry winter months.

Warm Compress: Applying a warm compress over your sinuses can provide relief by promoting blood circulation and easing congestion.

Elevated Sleep Position: Using an extra pillow or raising the head of your bed slightly can prevent mucus from pooling in your nasal passages while you sleep.

Hydration: Drinking plenty of fluids helps thin mucus and keeps your body hydrated, aiding in clearing congestion.

Spicy Foods: Foods with capsaicin, such as chili peppers, can temporarily relieve nasal congestion by causing a runny nose.

Nasal Strips: Adhesive nasal strips can help open up nasal passages by physically widening the nostrils.

Eucalyptus Oil: Adding a few drops of eucalyptus oil to hot water and inhaling the steam can provide relief due to its anti-inflammatory properties.

Avoid Irritants: Stay away from irritants like smoke, strong odors, and allergens that can worsen congestion.

Nettle Tea: Nettle tea contains natural antihistamines that can help reduce nasal congestion caused by allergies.

Remember, these remedies might work differently for each person, so it's important to find what works best for you. If nasal congestion persists or worsens, it's a good idea to consult a healthcare professional for further guidance.

5.3 The Role of Humidifiers in Reducing Nasal Congestion

Humidifiers play a significant role in alleviating nasal congestion by increasing the moisture levels in indoor air. When the air is dry, the mucus membranes in the nose can become dry and irritated, leading to congestion, discomfort, and even nosebleeds in some cases. Humidifiers work by releasing water vapor into the air, which helps maintain optimal humidity levels in indoor environments.

Nasal congestion often occurs due to various factors such as colds, allergies, sinus infections, and dry air. Dry air can further irritate the nasal passages, causing them to become inflamed and congested. By introducing moisture into the air through a humidifier, the nasal passages stay hydrated, promoting better respiratory function.

There are two main types of humidifiers: cool mist and warm mist. Cool mist humidifiers release room-temperature water vapor, making them suitable for year-round use. They are particularly beneficial in homes with children or pets, as there is no risk of accidental burns. Warm mist humidifiers, on the other hand, heat the water before releasing it as steam, which can be particularly soothing for congestion. However, they should be used with caution to prevent burns, especially around children.

It's important to note that while humidifiers are effective in reducing nasal congestion, their misuse can lead to problems such as mold and bacterial growth. To ensure safe and effective use, it's essential to follow the manufacturer's instructions for cleaning and maintaining the humidifier. Regular cleaning prevents the buildup of mold and bacteria in the water tank, which can be dispersed into the air and exacerbate respiratory issues.

In conclusion, humidifiers are valuable tools in reducing nasal congestion by increasing humidity levels and preventing the drying of nasal passages. Choosing the right type of humidifier and maintaining it properly can contribute to improved respiratory comfort, especially during dry seasons or when dealing with congestion-related ailments.

Chapter 6

Over-the-Counter Solutions for Snoring

Snoring can be disruptive for both the snorer and their sleeping partners. While there are numerous over-the-counter (OTC) solutions available to address snoring, it's important to note that their effectiveness can vary based on the underlying cause of the snoring. Here are some common OTC solutions:

Nasal Strips: These adhesive strips are applied to the outside of the nose and work by opening up the nasal passages, which can help reduce snoring caused by nasal congestion or a deviated septum.

Nasal Dilators: These are devices inserted into the nostrils to help keep the airways open, improving airflow and potentially reducing snoring.

Anti-Snoring Sprays: These sprays often contain natural oils or lubricants that aim to reduce vibrations in the throat, which can contribute to snoring. They are usually sprayed at the back of the throat before bed.

Throat Sprays: These sprays typically contain ingredients that help to lubricate and tone the tissues at the back of the throat, potentially reducing the vibrations that lead to snoring.

Oral Appliances: Some OTC oral devices are designed to reposition the jaw or tongue during sleep, which can help prevent airway obstruction and reduce snoring. These devices are often used for mild to moderate cases of snoring.

Positional Therapy Devices: These devices are worn during sleep and are designed to encourage sleeping in a specific position (such as sleeping on one's side), which can help prevent the relaxation of the throat muscles that lead to snoring.

Anti-Snoring Pillows: These pillows are designed to encourage sleeping in a particular position that promotes proper airway alignment and reduces snoring.

Homeopathic Remedies: Some OTC homeopathic products claim to reduce snoring through natural ingredients. However, the scientific evidence supporting their effectiveness is often limited.

Lifestyle Changes: While not direct OTC products, lifestyle changes such as weight loss, avoiding alcohol before bed, staying hydrated, and practicing good sleep hygiene can contribute to reducing snoring.

It's important to keep in mind that OTC solutions may not work for everyone, and their effectiveness can depend on the individual's unique snoring triggers. If snoring persists despite trying OTC solutions, or if it's accompanied by other symptoms like excessive daytime sleepiness, it's advisable to consult a healthcare professional. They can help identify the underlying cause of the snoring and recommend appropriate treatment options, which may include medical interventions or lifestyle changes.

6.1 Nasal Strips and Dilators for snoring prevention

Nasal strips and dilators are popular devices used for snoring prevention by improving nasal airflow and reducing the vibrations in the airway that cause snoring. They are non-invasive solutions that aim to alleviate snoring by addressing nasal congestion and airflow restrictions during sleep.

Nasal Strips:
Nasal strips are adhesive strips that are placed externally on the outside of the nose. They work by physically pulling open the nostrils, which helps to widen the nasal passages and improve airflow. The improved airflow can help reduce the resistance to breathing, which in turn can minimize the vibrations that lead to snoring.

Nasal strips are often made from flexible materials and have a spring-like quality that helps keep the nostrils open. They are relatively simple to use and can provide immediate relief for some individuals with minor snoring issues.

Nasal Dilators:
Nasal dilators are devices designed to be inserted directly into the nostrils. They work by gently expanding the nostrils from the inside, which has a similar effect to nasal strips—widening the nasal passages and allowing for better airflow. Nasal dilators come in various forms, including internal clips, cones, or plugs. Some dilators are made of soft, flexible materials, while others might be more rigid. Nasal dilators are generally well-tolerated and can be effective in cases where nasal congestion or structural issues contribute to snoring.

Effectiveness and Considerations:
Both nasal strips and dilators are most effective for individuals who snore due to nasal congestion, deviated septum, or other anatomical issues that obstruct airflow through

the nose. However, it's important to note that they might be less effective for snoring caused by issues in the throat or soft palate.

While these devices can provide relief, they are not a cure for sleep apnea or severe snoring conditions. If snoring is accompanied by other symptoms like excessive daytime sleepiness, choking during sleep, or witnessed pauses in breathing, it's essential to consult a healthcare professional. They can diagnose the underlying cause of the snoring and recommend appropriate treatment options.

It's also worth mentioning that individual experiences with nasal strips and dilators can vary. Some people find them very effective, while others may not experience significant improvement. It's often a matter of trying different products to find what works best for an individual's specific anatomy and snoring pattern.

In conclusion, nasal strips and dilators offer a non-invasive approach to addressing snoring by improving nasal airflow. They are particularly suitable for those whose snoring is related to nasal congestion or structural issues. However, consulting a medical professional is crucial for proper diagnosis and treatment, especially if snoring is indicative of a more serious sleep disorder.

6.2 Oral Sprays and Mouth Rinses for snoring solution

Oral sprays and mouth rinses have gained attention as potential solutions for snoring, offering a non-invasive approach to addressing this common issue. While there is ongoing research and development in this area, it's important to note that the effectiveness of these products can vary and may not completely eliminate snoring for everyone.

These products typically work by targeting the tissues in the throat and mouth that contribute to snoring. Snoring often occurs due to the narrowing of the airway during sleep, leading to vibrations in the soft tissues of the throat. Oral sprays and mouth rinses may contain various active ingredients designed to alleviate this narrowing and reduce the vibrations, thus diminishing the sound of snoring.

Common ingredients found in these products include:

Anti-Inflammatory Agents: Some oral sprays and mouth rinses contain anti-inflammatory compounds like chamomile, peppermint, or eucalyptus. These ingredients are believed to help reduce inflammation in the throat and airway tissues, potentially decreasing the likelihood of snoring.

Lubricants: Certain products include lubricating agents such as glycerin or xylitol. These substances aim to keep the tissues in the throat moist, which might help prevent them from sticking together and causing snoring sounds.

Tightening Agents: Some sprays contain ingredients like tannic acid or witch hazel, which are intended to tighten the tissues in the throat. This tightening effect could potentially reduce the vibration that leads to snoring.

Mild Anesthetics: A few products contain mild anesthetic agents like benzocaine. These substances may help numb the throat tissues, potentially reducing their tendency to vibrate and create snoring sounds.

Humectants: Humectants like hyaluronic acid might be included to keep the tissues hydrated and prevent them from becoming too relaxed during sleep.

It's important to note that individual responses to these products can vary widely. While some users might experience a noticeable reduction in snoring, others might find minimal to no effect. Additionally, the long-term safety and effectiveness of using oral sprays and mouth rinses for snoring are still subjects of ongoing research.

Before trying any of these products, it's a good idea to consult with a medical professional, especially if you have underlying health conditions. Snoring can sometimes be a symptom of more serious sleep-related disorders like sleep apnea, which require proper diagnosis and treatment.

In conclusion, while oral sprays and mouth rinses for snoring offer a non-invasive approach to addressing snoring, their effectiveness is not guaranteed for everyone. Individual experiences may vary, and it's important to approach these products with realistic expectations and in consultation with a healthcare provider.

6.3 Anti-Snoring Devices and Mouthguards for snoring prevention

Anti-snoring devices and mouthguards are designed to address the common issue of snoring during sleep. Snoring occurs when the flow of air through the mouth and nose is partially obstructed, causing the tissues in the throat to vibrate and produce the characteristic sound. These devices aim to alleviate or prevent snoring by maintaining open airways, improving airflow, and reducing the vibration of soft tissues.

Nasal Dilators: These are small devices that are inserted into the nostrils to help widen the nasal passages. By increasing the airflow through the nose, they can reduce the likelihood of mouth breathing, which is a common cause of snoring. Nasal dilators can be especially helpful for individuals whose snoring is primarily caused by nasal congestion or structural issues.

Tongue Stabilizing Devices (TSDs): TSDs are designed to keep the tongue in a forward position, preventing it from falling back and obstructing the throat during sleep. This helps maintain an open airway and reduces the chances of snoring. TSDs are particularly useful for individuals whose snoring is related to the tongue's position during sleep.

Mandibular Advancement Devices (MADs): MADs are perhaps the most common type of anti-snoring device. These devices resemble mouthguards and work by repositioning the lower jaw slightly forward during sleep. This adjustment helps prevent the collapse of the soft tissues at the back of the throat, which can cause snoring. MADs are customizable and can be obtained through dentists or over-the-counter options.

Continuous Positive Airway Pressure (CPAP) Machines: CPAP machines are commonly used to treat sleep apnea, a condition where breathing repeatedly stops and starts during sleep. However, they can also help prevent snoring. A CPAP machine delivers a continuous stream of air through a mask, maintaining positive pressure in the airway and preventing its collapse. While effective, CPAP machines can be cumbersome for some users.

Positional Therapy Devices: Snoring often worsens when an individual sleeps on their back, as this position can cause the tongue and soft palate to collapse to the back of the throat. Positional therapy devices are designed to prevent back sleeping, usually through the use of specialized pillows or wearable devices that provide discomfort if the user attempts to sleep on their back.

Palatal Implants: This is a more invasive option where small rods are inserted into the soft palate to stiffen it. This reduces the vibrations that lead to snoring. It's a procedure that requires medical intervention and is generally reserved for cases where other non-invasive options have failed.

It's important to note that the effectiveness of these devices varies from person to person. Snoring can be caused by various factors such as obesity, nasal congestion, sleep position, alcohol consumption, and more. Consulting a healthcare professional before using any anti-snoring device is recommended to determine the underlying cause of snoring and the most suitable solution. Additionally, some devices may cause discomfort

or have potential side effects, so proper guidance
is crucial.

Chapter 7

Seeking Professional Help for Snoring

Snoring can be disruptive to both the snorer and their sleep partner, often indicating an underlying issue that may require professional attention. Seeking help for snoring involves a step-by-step approach that begins with understanding the causes and severity of the problem.

Self-awareness: Start by identifying the frequency and intensity of your snoring. Keep a sleep diary noting factors like sleep position, alcohol or medication consumption, and daytime tiredness.

Lifestyle adjustments: Certain lifestyle changes can alleviate mild snoring. Losing weight, avoiding alcohol and sedatives before bedtime, maintaining a regular sleep schedule, and sleeping on your side might help reduce snoring.

Positional therapy: If your snoring worsens when sleeping on your back, you can use special pillows or devices that encourage sleeping on your side.

Nasal congestion: Addressing nasal congestion through saline sprays, decongestants, or nasal strips can help improve airflow and reduce snoring.

Sleep hygiene: Practicing good sleep hygiene, such as creating a comfortable sleep environment, can contribute to better sleep quality and potentially lessen snoring.

Medical evaluation: If lifestyle changes don't yield significant improvements, consult a healthcare professional. A primary care physician or an otolaryngologist (ear, nose, and throat specialist) can evaluate your condition.

Sleep study: In some cases, a sleep study (polysomnography) might be recommended. This involves spending a night at a sleep center where your sleep patterns, breathing, and snoring are monitored. This can help diagnose conditions like obstructive sleep apnea (OSA).

Treatment options:

Continuous Positive Airway Pressure (CPAP): If diagnosed with OSA, CPAP therapy might be prescribed. This involves wearing a mask that delivers a continuous stream of air, keeping the airways open during sleep.
Oral appliances: These devices are designed to reposition the jaw and tongue to prevent airway obstruction. They are particularly useful for mild to moderate OSA cases.
Surgery: Surgical options may be considered if structural issues like deviated septum or enlarged tonsils are causing the snoring.
Laser treatments: Some non-invasive laser therapies can help tighten or remove excess tissue in the throat, reducing snoring.

Follow-up: Regularly communicate with your healthcare provider to discuss progress and adjust treatment if needed.

Remember, seeking professional help is crucial if snoring is accompanied by symptoms like excessive daytime sleepiness, gasping for air during sleep, or choking sensations. Addressing snoring not only improves sleep quality but also promotes overall health and well-being.

7.1 When to Consult a Healthcare Professional

Consulting a healthcare professional is essential for various health concerns. Some situations that warrant seeking medical advice include:

Severe or Prolonged Symptoms: If you experience severe or prolonged symptoms, such as intense pain, high fever, persistent vomiting, or difficulty breathing, it's crucial to consult a healthcare professional.

New or Worsening Symptoms: If you notice new symptoms or your existing symptoms worsen over time, it's a sign to seek medical attention. This could indicate an underlying health issue.

Chronic Conditions: If you have a chronic health condition, regular consultations with a healthcare professional are necessary to manage and monitor your condition effectively.

Medication Management: When starting a new medication or experiencing adverse reactions to current medications, consulting a healthcare professional can help ensure proper dosages and minimize risks.

Infections: In the case of infections, such as urinary tract infections, respiratory infections, or skin infections, timely treatment is crucial to prevent complications.

Injuries: For injuries like fractures, deep cuts, head injuries, or injuries that cause severe pain, seeking medical attention is essential for proper assessment and treatment.

Mental Health Concerns: If you or someone you know is struggling with mental health issues like depression, anxiety, or suicidal thoughts, reaching out to a mental health professional or healthcare provider is vital.

Preventive Care: Regular check-ups and screenings can help detect potential health problems early. Consult your healthcare professional for recommended screenings based on your age, gender, and medical history.

Women's Health: Women should consult healthcare professionals for gynecological issues, family planning, and pregnancy-related concerns.

Children's Health: Children should see healthcare professionals for regular check-ups, vaccinations, growth monitoring, and developmental assessments.

Allergic Reactions: If you experience severe allergic reactions, such as difficulty breathing, swelling, or hives, seek immediate medical attention.

Unexplained Weight Changes: Sudden or unexplained weight loss or gain could be indicative of underlying health issues that need professional evaluation.

Chronic Pain: Persistent pain that affects your daily life should be discussed with a healthcare professional to identify its cause and develop an appropriate management plan.

Digestive Issues: Persistent digestive problems like chronic diarrhea, constipation, or blood in stool require medical evaluation.

Unusual Changes: Any sudden, unusual changes in your body, such as skin moles changing shape or color, should be examined by a healthcare professional.

Remember, it's better to consult a healthcare professional and receive appropriate guidance rather than trying to self-diagnose or self-treat potentially serious health issues. Your healthcare provider can offer personalized advice and treatment options based on your specific circumstances.

7.2 Common Medical Conditions Contributing to Snoring

Here is an in-depth exploration of common medical conditions that can contribute to snoring:

Obstructive Sleep Apnea (OSA): This is one of the leading causes of snoring. OSA occurs when the upper airway becomes partially or completely blocked during sleep, leading to pauses in breathing. The resulting decrease in oxygen levels prompts the body to wake briefly, often with loud snoring, to restore normal breathing.

Nasal Congestion: Conditions like allergies, colds, or sinus infections can cause nasal congestion and swelling of the nasal passages.

This can restrict the airflow, making it more difficult to breathe through the nose and leading to snoring as a result.

Obesity: Excess weight, especially around the neck, can put pressure on the throat muscles and narrow the airway. This can lead to vibrations in the throat tissues during sleep, resulting in snoring.

Enlarged Tonsils and Adenoids: In children and some adults, enlarged tonsils and adenoids can obstruct the airway, making it harder to breathe freely during sleep. This obstruction can lead to snoring.

Deviated Septum: A deviated septum is when the cartilage dividing the two nostrils is crooked or off-center. This can cause airflow irregularities, leading to snoring.

Hypothyroidism: An underactive thyroid gland can lead to weight gain and fluid retention, which may contribute to snoring by narrowing the airway.

GERD (Gastroesophageal Reflux Disease): Acid reflux can cause stomach acid to flow back into the throat while lying down, irritating the throat tissues and potentially causing snoring.

Neuromuscular Conditions: Certain conditions, such as muscular dystrophy, can weaken the muscles in the throat and tongue, leading to increased relaxation during sleep and contributing to snoring.

Alcohol and Sedative Use: Consuming alcohol or sedative medications before bedtime can relax the muscles in the throat excessively, leading to snoring.

Aging: With age, the muscles in the throat can lose tone and become floppier, increasing the likelihood of snoring.

Pregnancy: Hormonal changes and weight gain during pregnancy can lead to nasal congestion and weight around the neck, both of which can contribute to snoring.

Acromegaly: This rare hormonal disorder causes the body to produce excessive growth hormone, leading to enlargement of facial bones, including the jaw. An enlarged jaw can create a smaller airway space, potentially causing snoring.

Cushing's Syndrome: This disorder results from high levels of cortisol, which can lead to weight gain and fluid retention. These factors may increase the risk of snoring.

It's important to note that snoring itself might not always indicate a serious medical condition, but it's worth addressing if it's causing disruptions to sleep quality or if it's a symptom of an underlying health issue. If snoring is a persistent problem, consulting a healthcare professional or a sleep specialist is recommended for accurate diagnosis and appropriate treatment.

7.3 Diagnostic Tests and Assessments for Snoring

Diagnostic tests and assessments for snoring play a crucial role in understanding the underlying causes and severity of the condition. These evaluations aid in determining appropriate treatment strategies and identifying potential health risks associated with snoring. Several diagnostic methods are commonly utilized to assess snoring:

Medical History Review: The initial step involves discussing the patient's medical history, sleep patterns, lifestyle, and any associated symptoms. This helps in identifying potential risk factors and narrowing down the possible causes of snoring.

Physical Examination: A comprehensive physical examination may reveal anatomical factors that contribute to snoring. This includes assessing the nasal passages, throat, mouth, and neck for abnormalities or structural issues such as enlarged tonsils, deviated septum, or obesity.

Questionnaires and Sleep Logs: Patients may be asked to fill out questionnaires or maintain sleep logs to track their sleep patterns and snoring episodes over a period. These logs provide valuable insights into the frequency and severity of snoring, along with potential triggers.

Sleep Studies (Polysomnography): Polysomnography is a comprehensive sleep study conducted in a sleep laboratory or at home. It monitors various physiological parameters during sleep, including brain activity, eye movement, muscle activity, heart rate, respiratory effort, and blood oxygen levels. This test helps diagnose sleep disorders such as obstructive sleep apnea (OSA) which is often associated with loud snoring.

Home Sleep Apnea Testing (HSAT): For individuals with a high likelihood of having obstructive sleep apnea, portable devices can be used to conduct sleep studies at home. These devices are less comprehensive than polysomnography but provide a convenient and cost-effective means of assessing snoring and sleep apnea.

Nasal Endoscopy: A nasal endoscopy involves inserting a thin, flexible tube with a camera into the nasal passages to evaluate the upper airway for any obstructions, abnormalities, or anatomical issues.

Acoustic Analysis: Acoustic analysis involves recording snoring sounds and analyzing their frequency, intensity, and pattern. This can offer insights into the characteristics of snoring and its potential causes.

Imaging Studies: Imaging techniques like X-rays, CT scans, or MRI scans can provide detailed images of the upper airway and help identify structural abnormalities that contribute to snoring.

Sleep Apps and Wearables: Some smartphone apps and wearable devices are designed to track sleep and snoring patterns. While these may not provide clinical-grade accuracy, they can offer individuals a basic understanding of their sleep quality and snoring behavior.

It's important to note that a combination of these diagnostic methods may be employed to get a comprehensive understanding of the factors contributing to snoring. The choice of tests depends on the patient's symptoms, medical history, and suspected underlying causes. Seeking guidance from a healthcare professional, particularly a sleep specialist, is essential to determine the most appropriate diagnostic approach and subsequent treatment plan.

7.4 Treatment Options: CPAP Machines, Oral Appliances, and Surgical Interventions

CPAP Machines (Continuous Positive Airway Pressure): CPAP machines are devices that deliver a constant stream of air pressure to keep the airways open during sleep. They are commonly used to treat sleep apnea, a condition where breathing pauses repeatedly during sleep. CPAP therapy helps maintain steady breathing and prevents interruptions.

Oral Appliances: Oral appliances are custom-made devices, often similar to mouthguards or dental splints, that are worn during sleep. They are designed to reposition the jaw and tongue to prevent the airway from becoming obstructed. Oral appliances are another treatment option for sleep apnea, especially for those who prefer an alternative to CPAP machines.

Surgical Interventions: Surgical treatments are considered for severe cases of sleep apnea that do not respond well to non-invasive methods. Surgical options may include procedures to remove excess tissue from the throat, reshape the jaw, or adjust the positioning of certain structures to improve airflow. These interventions are typically recommended when other treatments have not been effective.

Keep in mind that the choice of treatment depends on the severity of the condition, the patient's preferences, and other individual factors. It's important to consult a medical professional to determine the most suitable treatment approach for your specific situation.

treatment options for sleep apnea:

CPAP Machines (Continuous Positive Airway Pressure):
CPAP therapy is a common and effective treatment for obstructive sleep apnea (OSA). A CPAP machine delivers a continuous stream of air pressure through a mask worn over the nose and/or mouth. This air pressure prevents the airway from collapsing during sleep, thereby ensuring uninterrupted breathing. CPAP machines come in various styles, including standard CPAP, APAP (Auto-Adjusting Positive Airway Pressure), and BiPAP (Bilevel Positive Airway Pressure), each catering to different needs.

Oral Appliances (Mandibular Advancement Devices):
Oral appliances are designed to reposition the lower jaw and tongue to keep the airway open during sleep. These devices are often used to treat mild to moderate cases of obstructive sleep apnea, especially for individuals who cannot tolerate CPAP therapy. Dentists with expertise in sleep medicine create custom-fitted devices that suit the patient's mouth structure and needs.

Surgical Interventions:
Surgical options are considered when other treatments are ineffective or inappropriate. There are several surgical procedures available:

Uvulopalatopharyngoplasty (UPPP): This surgery removes excess tissue from the throat, such as the uvula and parts of the soft palate, to widen the airway.

Genioglossus Advancement (GA): In this procedure, a small part of the lower jawbone is repositioned to prevent the tongue from collapsing into the airway.

Maxillomandibular Advancement (MMA): This surgery repositions the upper and lower jaw to enlarge the airway. It's usually reserved for severe cases of sleep apnea.

Inspire Therapy: A newer approach involves implanting a device that stimulates the hypoglossal nerve to prevent airway collapse during sleep.

Laser-Assisted Uvulopalatoplasty (LAUP): Laser technology is used to remove or reshape excess tissue in the throat.

Nasal Surgery: Correcting structural issues in the nose, such as a deviated septum, can help improve airflow.

It's important to note that treatment recommendations should be made based on an individual's specific diagnosis, severity of sleep apnea, overall health, and personal preferences.

A sleep specialist or medical professional should be consulted to determine the most suitable treatment plan. Additionally, lifestyle changes such as weight loss, positional therapy, and avoiding alcohol and sedatives before bedtime can complement these treatments and enhance their effectiveness.

Chapter 8

Partner Support and Communication

Partner Support and Communication is a critical aspect of any collaborative endeavor or business relationship. It involves establishing effective channels and strategies to facilitate clear and consistent communication between partners, as well as providing the necessary assistance and resources to ensure the success of the partnership.

Effective partner support and communication begin with a solid foundation built on mutual understanding, shared goals, and a well-defined partnership agreement. This agreement should outline each partner's responsibilities, expectations, and contributions, serving as a reference point for the partnership's activities.

Clear channels of communication are essential to keep partners informed about project progress, changes in strategy, or any potential challenges. Regular meetings, whether in-person or virtual, help partners stay aligned and updated on the partnership's direction. These meetings provide an opportunity to discuss achievements, address concerns, and brainstorm solutions collaboratively.

In addition to formal meetings, maintaining an open line of communication through various mediums, such as emails, instant messaging, and phone calls, enhances real-time interaction. This enables partners to share information, ask questions, and seek clarification promptly, fostering a sense of transparency and trust.

Effective partner support involves being responsive to partners' needs and challenges. This might include providing technical assistance, offering training sessions, or allocating resources to help partners overcome obstacles. An effective support system ensures that partners feel valued and empowered to contribute effectively to the partnership's goals.

Flexibility in communication styles and methods is crucial, as different partners may have varying preferences or cultural nuances that influence how they communicate. Being adaptable and respectful of these differences can help prevent misunderstandings and build stronger relationships.

To sum up, successful partner support and communication require a combination of clear expectations, consistent interaction, timely information sharing, and a willingness to provide assistance when needed. When executed effectively, these elements contribute to the overall success of the partnership by fostering collaboration, trust, and a shared sense of purpose.

8.1 Understanding the Impact of Snoring on Relationships

Snoring can have a profound impact on relationships, extending beyond its mere acoustic disturbance. The consistent noise disrupts sleep patterns, leading to sleep deprivation and fatigue for both the snorer and their partner. This physical toll can trigger irritability, mood swings, and decreased cognitive function, which in turn strain communication and emotional connection.

Furthermore, the non-snoring partner's sleep disruption can evoke feelings of resentment and frustration. They may experience a sense of helplessness in addressing the issue, leading to a breakdown in intimacy and understanding. Over time, this can erode the foundation of trust and emotional closeness, potentially leading to conflicts and emotional detachment.

The impact extends beyond just the bedroom. Sleep-deprived individuals are less likely to engage in social activities, and the lack of energy and focus may limit their involvement in shared hobbies or responsibilities. This can lead to a sense of isolation and reduced quality time spent together.

Addressing snoring-related relationship issues requires open and honest communication. Couples need to work together to find solutions, whether through lifestyle changes, medical interventions, or separate sleeping arrangements. Seeking professional help, such as consulting a sleep specialist, can provide valuable insights and potential remedies.

In conclusion, the impact of snoring on relationships is multifaceted. From disrupting sleep and triggering emotional strain to affecting intimacy and shared activities, it's crucial for couples to acknowledge and address the issue together in order to preserve and strengthen their bond.

8.2 Strategies for Open Communication about Snoring

Open communication about snoring can be crucial for maintaining a healthy relationship and addressing potential underlying health concerns. Here are some strategies for engaging in open communication about snoring:

Choose the Right Time and Place: Find a comfortable and private setting where both you and your partner can talk openly without distractions or interruptions.

Use "I" Statements: Frame your concerns using "I" statements, such as "I've noticed that your snoring has been affecting my sleep," instead of blaming or accusing.

Express Concern, Not Criticism: Express your concern for their well-being rather than criticizing or making them feel embarrassed about their snoring.

Listen Actively: Give your partner the opportunity to share their perspective on the issue. Active listening shows that you value their thoughts and feelings.

Be Empathetic: Acknowledge that snoring can be embarrassing or frustrating for them as well. Show empathy for any discomfort they might be experiencing.

Discuss Health Implications: Mention that snoring could be a sign of an underlying health issue, like sleep apnea, which can have serious consequences if left untreated.

Offer Support: Suggest that both of you work together to find a solution. Offer your support in seeking medical advice or trying remedies.

Research Together: Explore possible causes of snoring and potential solutions together. This collaborative approach can foster a sense of teamwork.

Discuss Lifestyle Changes: Talk about lifestyle factors that might contribute to snoring, such as weight, alcohol consumption, or sleep position. Discussing changes can be less confrontational if you both commit to healthier habits.

Consider Professional Help: If snoring persists, recommend consulting a healthcare professional, such as an ear, nose, and throat specialist or a sleep specialist. This shows your commitment to finding a solution.

Explore Treatment Options: If sleep apnea is suspected, discuss treatment options like Continuous Positive Airway Pressure (CPAP) therapy or lifestyle adjustments with a medical professional.

Use Humor Wisely: Using humor can help lighten the mood, but be cautious not to belittle or trivialize the issue.

Reinforce Positives: Acknowledge and celebrate any progress or positive changes that occur as a result of your open communication and joint efforts.

Remember, open communication is about fostering understanding and finding solutions together. Approach the conversation with kindness and a genuine desire to improve the situation for both of you.

8.3 Supporting Each Other in Finding Solutions

Supporting each other in finding solutions is a crucial aspect of effective collaboration and problem-solving. When individuals come together to address challenges, their combined perspectives, skills, and insights can lead to innovative and comprehensive solutions.

Effective support involves several key elements:

Active Listening: To understand each other's viewpoints and concerns, active listening is essential. This means giving your full attention, asking clarifying questions, and showing empathy to ensure everyone's voice is heard and understood.

Open Communication: Creating an environment where everyone feels comfortable sharing their ideas, opinions, and suggestions is vital. Open communication promotes transparency and encourages the exploration of diverse solutions.

Respect for Diversity: Individuals bring unique backgrounds, experiences, and expertise to the table. Respecting this diversity fosters a rich pool of ideas, as different perspectives can lead to novel approaches.

Collaborative Problem Definition: Before jumping into solutions, collaboratively define and understand the problem at hand. This shared understanding ensures that efforts are aligned and focused on the right issues.

Brainstorming: Encourage brainstorming sessions where all participants can freely propose ideas without judgment. This creative phase allows for the generation of a wide range of possible solutions.

Critical Evaluation: After brainstorming, evaluate the proposed solutions critically. Discuss the potential pros and cons of each approach, considering feasibility, resources, and potential outcomes.

Consensus Building: Aim for consensus on the chosen solution, taking into account the concerns and preferences of all participants. This ensures that everyone is invested in the decision-making process.

Allocation of Responsibilities: Clearly define roles and responsibilities for implementing the chosen solution. Each person's strengths and expertise can be leveraged to contribute effectively.

Regular Updates: Maintain open lines of communication throughout the solution implementation process. Regular updates help track progress, address challenges, and make necessary adjustments.

Adaptability and Flexibility: Be open to modifying the chosen solution if new information arises or if initial attempts don't yield the expected results. Adaptability is key to finding the most effective approach.

Recognition and Appreciation: Acknowledge and appreciate each individual's contributions and efforts. Recognizing the value of everyone's input fosters a positive and collaborative atmosphere.

Learning from Mistakes: If a solution doesn't work as intended, view it as an opportunity to learn and improve. Analyze what went wrong and apply those lessons to future problem-solving endeavors.

By supporting each other through active collaboration, open communication, and a shared commitment to finding effective solutions, teams and individuals can navigate challenges with resilience and creativity.

Chapter 9

Natural Remedies for Snoring

Natural remedies for snoring. Snoring can be caused by various factors, such as nasal congestion, obesity, sleep position, or even lifestyle habits. While it's important to address the underlying causes, here are some natural remedies that might help reduce or alleviate snoring:

Lifestyle Changes:

Weight Management: Losing excess weight, especially around the neck area, can help reduce snoring as it decreases pressure on the airways.
Sleep Position: Sleeping on your back can worsen snoring. Try sleeping on your side to keep your airways open.
Healthy Diet: Consuming a balanced diet rich in fruits, vegetables, and lean proteins can

contribute to overall better sleep and potentially reduce snoring.

Nasal Congestion Relief:

Steam Inhalation: Inhaling steam from a bowl of hot water can help open nasal passages and reduce congestion.

Nasal Strips: External nasal strips can help widen the nostrils, making it easier to breathe and reducing snoring.

Humidification:

Humidifiers: Adding moisture to the air in your bedroom can prevent the throat and nasal passages from becoming dry, reducing the likelihood of snoring.

Herbal Remedies:

Peppermint Oil: Peppermint oil has anti-inflammatory properties that can help alleviate nasal congestion. You can inhale its aroma before sleeping or apply a diluted solution to your chest.

Throat Exercises:

Tongue and Throat Exercises: Strengthening the muscles in your tongue and throat can help prevent them from collapsing and causing snoring. For example, pressing the tip of your tongue against the roof of your mouth and sliding it backward several times a day can be beneficial.

Avoiding Alcohol and Sedatives:

Alcohol and sedatives: These substances relax the muscles in your throat, which can contribute to snoring. Avoid consuming them close to bedtime.

Hydration:

Adequate Hydration: Staying hydrated helps keep the tissues in your throat from becoming sticky and causing vibrations that lead to snoring.

It's important to note that individual results may vary, and not all remedies might work for everyone. If snoring persists despite trying these natural remedies, it's recommended to consult a medical professional. Chronic snoring could be a sign of a more serious underlying condition, such as sleep apnea, that requires medical attention.

9.1 Herbal Supplements and Essential Oils for snoring treatment

Snoring is a common condition caused by the vibration of tissues in the throat and nose during sleep. While there's limited scientific evidence supporting the effectiveness of herbal supplements and essential oils for treating snoring, some people find them to be helpful. Keep in mind that individual responses can vary, and it's always a good idea to consult a healthcare professional before trying any new treatment.

Peppermint Essential Oil: Peppermint oil has anti-inflammatory properties that might help reduce inflammation in the airways and improve breathing. You can dilute a few drops of peppermint oil in a carrier oil (like coconut oil) and apply it to your chest or the bottoms of your feet before bed.

Eucalyptus Essential Oil: Eucalyptus oil is known for its ability to open up airways and promote easier breathing. Similar to peppermint oil, you can dilute a few drops of eucalyptus oil and apply it topically or use it in a diffuser in your bedroom.

Lavender Essential Oil: Lavender oil is known for its calming and relaxing effects. While it might not directly address snoring, using lavender oil in a diffuser could potentially promote better sleep quality, which might indirectly help with snoring.

Thyme Essential Oil: Thyme oil has antibacterial and antiseptic properties. It could be used to maintain a healthy respiratory system, which might reduce congestion and snoring. Dilute and apply topically, or use it in a diffuser.

Herbal Tea Blends: Certain herbal teas, like chamomile or peppermint, might help soothe throat tissues and promote relaxation. Warm tea before bed could contribute to a more peaceful sleep, potentially reducing snoring.

Ginger: Ginger has anti-inflammatory properties that could reduce inflammation in the airways. You can consume ginger in tea or add it to your diet. It's worth noting that excessive ginger intake could have side effects, so moderation is key.

Honey: Honey has been used for its potential anti-inflammatory properties and soothing effects on the throat. Mixing a teaspoon of honey in warm water or herbal tea before bed might help reduce irritation in the airways.

Nasal Irrigation with Saline Solution: While not an essential oil or supplement, using a saline solution to rinse the nasal passages might help clear congestion and improve airflow, potentially reducing snoring.

Remember, snoring can also be caused by factors like obesity, sleep position, alcohol consumption, and sleep apnea. Lifestyle changes, such as maintaining a healthy weight, avoiding alcohol before bed, and sleeping on your side, can also contribute to reducing snoring. If snoring persists or is accompanied by other symptoms like daytime fatigue, it's important to consult a medical professional for a proper diagnosis and treatment plan.

9.2 Breathing Exercises and Yoga Techniques for snoring treatment

Here are some in-depth breathing exercises and yoga techniques that can help with snoring treatment:

Pranayama Techniques:

Nadi Shodhana (Alternate Nostril Breathing): Sit in a comfortable position, close your right nostril with your right thumb, and inhale deeply through your left nostril. Then, close your left nostril with your right ring finger and release the right nostril. Exhale slowly and deeply. Repeat the process, alternating nostrils. This technique helps balance the flow of breath and promotes better sleep.

Bhramari (Bee Breath): Close your eyes and inhale deeply. As you exhale, produce a humming sound like a bee by gently closing your ears with your thumbs and placing your index fingers over your closed eyes. The vibrations from the humming have a soothing effect on the nervous system and can help reduce snoring tendencies.
Yoga Asanas:

Ujjayi Pranayama (Victorious Breath): This involves breathing through the nose while slightly constricting the back of your throat. It's often used during yoga asanas to calm the mind and regulate breathing patterns, which can indirectly help with snoring.
Simhasana (Lion Pose): Kneel down with your hands on your thighs. Inhale deeply through your nose and open your mouth wide, sticking out your tongue as far as possible while exhaling forcefully. Roar like a lion. This exercise helps strengthen the throat muscles and may reduce the likelihood of snoring.
Lifestyle Changes:

Weight Management: Maintaining a healthy weight reduces the pressure on your airways, which can help prevent snoring.

Sleep Position: Sleeping on your back often worsens snoring. Try sleeping on your side instead to keep your airways open.

Avoid Alcohol and Sedatives: These substances can relax the muscles in your throat, contributing to snoring.

Hydration: Staying hydrated helps keep the tissues in your throat from becoming sticky and causing vibrations that lead to snoring.

Mindfulness and Relaxation:

Meditation: Practicing meditation can reduce stress and promote better sleep, which in turn can help with snoring.

Progressive Muscle Relaxation: This technique involves tensing and then releasing each muscle group in your body, promoting overall relaxation and potentially reducing snoring tendencies.

It's important to note that while these techniques can be beneficial, chronic snoring might be caused by underlying medical conditions such as sleep apnea. If snoring persists despite trying these techniques, it's recommended to consult a healthcare professional for a proper diagnosis and personalized treatment plan.

9.3 Lifestyle Habits for Better Sleep Hygiene as a natural remedy for snoring treatment

Here are some lifestyle habits that contribute to better sleep hygiene and can serve as a natural remedy for snoring treatment:

Maintain a Consistent Sleep Schedule: Going to bed and waking up at the same time every day helps regulate your body's internal clock, improving sleep quality and reducing snoring.

Create a Comfortable Sleep Environment: Ensure your bedroom is conducive to sleep by keeping it dark, quiet, and at a comfortable temperature. Using earplugs and blackout curtains can be helpful.

Invest in a Supportive Mattress and Pillows: A comfortable and supportive sleeping surface can help keep your airways open and minimize snoring.

Practice Relaxation Techniques: Engage in relaxation exercises like deep breathing, meditation, or yoga before bedtime to alleviate stress and tension that can contribute to snoring.

Limit Electronic Devices Before Bed: The blue light emitted by screens can interfere with your body's production of melatonin, a hormone that regulates sleep. Try to avoid screens at least an hour before sleeping.

Watch Your Diet: Avoid heavy meals, caffeine, and alcohol close to bedtime. These substances can relax your throat muscles and lead to snoring.

Stay Hydrated: Drink plenty of water throughout the day, but reduce your intake in the evening to minimize the likelihood of excess fluid in your throat that could cause snoring.

Maintain a Healthy Weight: Carrying excess weight, especially around your neck, can put pressure on your airways and increase the likelihood of snoring. Regular exercise and a balanced diet can help manage weight.

Sleep on Your Side: Sleeping on your back can cause your tongue and soft palate to collapse to the back of your throat, obstructing airflow and causing snoring. Try sleeping on your side instead.

Elevate Your Head: Using an extra pillow or raising the head of your bed slightly can help keep your airways open and reduce snoring.

Remember that while these lifestyle habits can certainly contribute to reducing snoring, the effectiveness may vary from person to person. If snoring persists or is causing significant sleep disruption, it's important to consult a healthcare professional for a thorough evaluation and personalized recommendations.

Chapter 10

Snoring in Children

Snoring in children can be caused by various factors. Common causes include enlarged tonsils or adenoids, which can obstruct the airway during sleep. Allergies, colds, or sinus infections might also contribute. Obesity can lead to excess throat tissue, narrowing the airway. In some cases, structural issues like a deviated septum could be at play.

Persistent snoring might indicate sleep apnea, a condition where breathing stops and starts during sleep. Sleep apnea can affect a child's sleep quality, leading to daytime sleepiness, difficulty concentrating, and behavioral problems.

It's crucial to consult a pediatrician if your child snores regularly. The doctor may recommend a sleep study to diagnose any underlying sleep disorders. Treatment options range from addressing underlying causes like allergies or infections, to surgical interventions like tonsillectomy or adenoidectomy. Lifestyle changes such as weight management and adjusting sleep position may also help alleviate snoring in children.

10.1 Common Causes and Concerns for Childhood Snoring

Childhood snoring can be attributed to various factors, with some being more common and concerning than others. Here, we'll delve into an in-depth exploration of the common causes and concerns associated with childhood snoring:

Enlarged Tonsils and Adenoids: One of the leading causes of childhood snoring is the enlargement of tonsils and adenoids. These lymphoid tissues located in the throat can obstruct the airway during sleep, leading to snoring. This concern is often addressed through surgical removal if it becomes persistent and affects the child's quality of sleep.

Nasal Congestion and Allergies: Children with chronic nasal congestion or allergies may experience snoring due to the narrowing of their nasal passages. Swollen nasal tissues hinder the smooth passage of air, resulting in snoring. Addressing the underlying allergies or congestion can alleviate this issue.

Obesity: Childhood obesity is on the rise and has been linked to various health problems, including snoring. Excess weight can lead to fatty deposits in the throat, narrowing the airway and causing snoring during sleep.

Sleep Position: Sleeping on the back can cause the tongue and soft palate to collapse to the back of the throat, partially blocking the airway and causing snoring. Encouraging a different sleep position might help reduce snoring.

Genetic Predisposition: Genetics can play a role in determining the anatomy of a child's airway. Children with a family history of snoring or sleep apnea may be more prone to snoring due to inherited traits that affect their airway structure.

Neuromuscular Factors: Some children might have weakened muscle tone in the throat and tongue, making it more likely for these tissues to collapse and cause snoring during sleep.

Sleep Apnea: While snoring is common, chronic and loud snoring could be indicative of a more serious condition known as sleep apnea. Sleep apnea occurs when the airway becomes completely blocked, causing the child to momentarily stop breathing during sleep. This can lead to disrupted sleep patterns and even affect cognitive development if left untreated.

GERD (Gastroesophageal Reflux Disease): GERD can cause stomach acid to flow back into the throat during sleep, leading to irritation and inflammation. This can cause snoring or exacerbate existing snoring issues.

Craniofacial Abnormalities: Certain congenital conditions or abnormalities in the structure of the face, jaw, or airway can contribute to snoring in children. These may require specialized medical attention.

Secondhand Smoke Exposure: Exposure to secondhand smoke can lead to airway inflammation and increased mucus production, both of which can contribute to snoring.

Environmental Factors: Factors such as dry air in the sleeping environment or the use of certain bedding materials can contribute to nasal congestion and subsequently lead to snoring.

It's important to note that occasional snoring is relatively common in children and might not always indicate a serious issue. However, persistent and loud snoring that affects the child's sleep quality or is accompanied by other symptoms like gasping for air during sleep, daytime sleepiness, behavioral problems, or difficulty concentrating should be evaluated by a medical professional. A proper diagnosis will help determine the underlying cause and guide appropriate treatment, ensuring the child's overall health and well-being.

10.2 Identifying Sleep Disorders in Children

Identifying sleep disorders in children is a crucial aspect of their overall health and development. Sleep disorders can have a significant impact on a child's physical, cognitive, and emotional well-being. In-depth evaluation involves several key considerations:

Symptom Recognition: Recognizing common symptoms such as difficulty falling asleep, frequent nighttime awakenings, snoring, gasping for air during sleep, bedwetting, restless legs, and excessive daytime sleepiness is essential. These symptoms could indicate various sleep disorders like sleep apnea, insomnia, restless leg syndrome, or parasomnias.

Medical History: Obtaining a detailed medical history from the child's parents or caregivers is crucial. Information about the child's sleep patterns, bedtime routines, and any medical conditions or medications that might affect sleep is valuable.

Sleep Diary: Asking parents to maintain a sleep diary can provide valuable insights into the child's sleep patterns and daily routines. This can help identify trends or triggers contributing to sleep issues.

Parental Observations: Parents may provide information about the child's behavior during sleep, such as snoring, breathing pauses, sleepwalking, or night terrors. This can help in diagnosing specific sleep disorders.

Physical Examination: Conducting a thorough physical examination can reveal signs of sleep disorders, such as enlarged tonsils or adenoids, which can contribute to sleep apnea.

Polysomnography (Sleep Study): In some cases, a sleep study may be recommended. This involves monitoring the child's sleep patterns, brain activity, breathing, heart rate, and movements during the night. It helps diagnose disorders like sleep apnea and narcolepsy.

Actigraphy: Actigraphy involves using a wrist-worn device to track the child's movements and sleep-wake patterns over a period. This can provide insights into the child's sleep quality and circadian rhythms.

Behavioral Assessment: For issues like insomnia or behavioral sleep problems, a behavioral assessment may be conducted to identify contributing factors and develop strategies to improve sleep hygiene.

Multidisciplinary Approach: In some cases, a team of specialists including pediatricians, sleep specialists, psychologists, and ear, nose, and throat (ENT) doctors may collaborate to diagnose and manage complex sleep disorders.

Treatment and Management: Once a sleep disorder is identified, an individualized treatment plan is developed. This may include lifestyle changes, behavioral interventions, medical treatments, or surgical options, depending on the specific disorder.

It's important to approach the identification of sleep disorders in children with sensitivity and care, considering the unique needs and developmental stages of each child. Early detection and intervention can lead to improved sleep quality, overall health, and well-being. If you suspect a sleep disorder in a child, consulting with a medical professional experienced in pediatric sleep medicine is recommended.

10.3 Treatment Options and Parental Support

Treatment options and parental support play a pivotal role in addressing various physical, emotional, and developmental challenges that children may face. In this discussion, we will delve into the in-depth aspects of treatment options and the crucial role that parental support plays in the overall well-being of children.

Treatment Options:

Medical Interventions: Depending on the specific condition, medical interventions can vary widely. This may include medications, surgeries, therapies, and assistive devices. Conditions like ADHD, autism, and physical disabilities often require tailored medical approaches to manage symptoms and enhance quality of life.

Therapies: Different types of therapies are available to address emotional, behavioral, and developmental concerns. Examples include cognitive-behavioral therapy (CBT), speech therapy, occupational therapy, and physical therapy. These therapies focus on improving specific skills and coping mechanisms.

Behavioral Interventions: For behavioral challenges, applied behavior analysis (ABA) and positive behavior support (PBS) are widely used. These approaches help children develop appropriate behaviors and social skills while reducing problem behaviors.

Educational Support: Many children require specialized education due to learning disabilities or developmental delays. Individualized Education Programs (IEPs) and 504 Plans in school settings provide tailored support and accommodations to help children thrive academically.

Alternative and Complementary Therapies: Some parents explore alternative therapies like art therapy, music therapy, or yoga to complement traditional treatments. It's important to consult with medical professionals before incorporating these methods.

Parental Support:

Emotional Support: Parents play a crucial role in providing emotional support, creating a safe space for their children to express their feelings, fears, and challenges. This support fosters a sense of security and trust.

Advocacy: Parents often need to advocate for their children within educational, medical, and social systems. This involves understanding their child's rights, collaborating with professionals, and ensuring their needs are met.

Education: Learning about their child's condition empowers parents to make informed decisions. Understanding treatment options, potential challenges, and available resources equips parents to provide the best possible care.

Consistency: Consistency in routines, expectations, and communication is crucial for children who may struggle with changes.

Predictable environments can help reduce anxiety and promote stability.

Self-Care: Parenting a child with special needs can be demanding. Parents must prioritize self-care to avoid burnout. Seeking support from support groups or therapists can be beneficial.

Collaboration: Partnering with medical professionals, therapists, teachers, and caregivers creates a comprehensive support network for the child. Collaborative efforts ensure that the child's needs are addressed holistically.

In conclusion, treatment options and parental support form a dynamic duo in promoting the well-being of children facing various challenges. While treatment options provide the necessary tools to manage conditions, parental support creates an environment of love, understanding, and empowerment, allowing these children to thrive and reach their full potential.

Chapter 11

Coping with Snoring-Related Sleep Deprivation

Coping with sleep deprivation due to snoring-related issues can be challenging, but there are several strategies you can consider to improve your sleep quality and overall well-being:

Identify the Underlying Cause: Understanding the root cause of snoring is essential. It can be due to various factors such as obesity, sleep position, allergies, or nasal congestion. Consult a healthcare professional to determine the cause and appropriate treatment.

Lifestyle Modifications:

Healthy Diet and Exercise: Maintaining a healthy weight through balanced nutrition and regular exercise can reduce snoring.
Sleep Hygiene: Establish a consistent sleep schedule, create a comfortable sleep environment, and limit screen time before bed.
Sleeping Position:

Side Sleeping: Sleeping on your side can help prevent the collapse of the airway and reduce snoring. You can use pillows to encourage this position.
Nasal Congestion Relief:

Nasal Strips: External adhesive strips can help widen nasal passages, enhancing airflow.
Nasal Irrigation: Rinsing the nasal passages with saline solution can clear congestion.
Avoid Alcohol and Sedatives: These substances relax the muscles in your throat, contributing to snoring. Limit their consumption, especially before bedtime.

Continuous Positive Airway Pressure (CPAP):

For severe cases of snoring and sleep apnea, a CPAP machine can provide a constant flow of air to keep the airway open.
Oral Appliances:

Some dental devices can help reposition the jaw and tongue to prevent snoring.
Medical Interventions:

Surgery: In extreme cases, surgical options such as uvulopalatopharyngoplasty (UPPP) or genioglossus advancement (GA) can be considered to address anatomical issues causing snoring.
Seek Support:

Talk to your partner about your struggles with snoring-related sleep deprivation. Their understanding can reduce any feelings of isolation.
Manage Daytime Fatigue:

Short naps during the day can help alleviate some of the sleep debt, but avoid long naps that might disrupt nighttime sleep further.

Relaxation Techniques:

Stress and anxiety can worsen snoring. Engage in relaxation practices like deep breathing, meditation, or yoga to reduce tension.

Consult a Professional:

If snoring persists despite trying these strategies, consult a sleep specialist. They can recommend appropriate diagnostic tests and treatment options.

Remember, each individual's situation is unique, so it's important to tailor your approach to your specific needs. Addressing snoring-related sleep deprivation requires patience and a comprehensive plan to improve both your sleep quality and overall health.

11.1 Understanding the Effects of Sleep Deprivation

Sleep deprivation can have profound effects on various aspects of human health and cognitive functioning. When individuals consistently do not get an adequate amount of sleep, it can lead to a range of physical, mental, and emotional consequences. Here is an in-depth exploration of the effects of sleep deprivation:

Cognitive Impairments: Sleep deprivation can severely impact cognitive functions such as attention, memory, decision-making, and problem-solving. The ability to focus on tasks diminishes, leading to reduced productivity and increased errors.

Emotional Disturbances: Lack of sleep can lead to mood swings, irritability, and heightened emotional sensitivity. It can also increase the risk of developing mood disorders like depression and anxiety.

Impaired Learning: Sleep plays a crucial role in memory consolidation, which is essential for effective learning. Depriving the brain of sufficient sleep impairs its ability to encode and retain new information.

Physical Health: Chronic sleep deprivation is associated with an increased risk of various health issues, including obesity, diabetes, cardiovascular diseases, and weakened immune function. These health concerns arise due to disrupted hormonal regulation and inflammation caused by insufficient sleep.

Metabolic Disruptions: Sleep deprivation can disrupt hormonal balance, leading to insulin resistance and irregularities in glucose metabolism. This can contribute to the development of type 2 diabetes.

Weight Gain: Poor sleep patterns can lead to changes in appetite-regulating hormones, causing an increased craving for high-calorie foods. This, combined with a slowed metabolism, can contribute to weight gain.

Weakened Immune System: During sleep, the immune system repairs and strengthens itself. Sleep deprivation compromises immune function, making individuals more susceptible to infections and illnesses.

Cardiovascular Consequences: Chronic sleep deprivation is linked to hypertension (high blood pressure), which is a major risk factor for heart disease and stroke.

Impact on Hormones: Sleep deprivation disrupts the balance of hormones like cortisol, which regulates stress response, and growth hormones, which aid in tissue repair and muscle growth.

Increased Accident Risk: Sleep-deprived individuals are more prone to accidents due to slower reaction times and impaired decision-making. This is especially critical for activities like driving or operating heavy machinery.

Affects on Mental Health: Prolonged sleep deprivation is associated with an increased risk of developing mental health disorders, including depression and anxiety. Sleep disturbances can exacerbate existing mental health conditions.

Reduced Libido: Sleep plays a role in regulating sex hormones, and sleep deprivation can lead to decreased libido and sexual dysfunction.

Aging Effects: Lack of sleep accelerates the aging process, manifesting in wrinkles, reduced skin elasticity, and cognitive decline often seen in older adults.

It's important to recognize that the effects of sleep deprivation can vary among individuals, and the severity of these effects depends on factors such as the duration and chronicity of sleep deprivation, age, genetics, and overall health. Prioritizing healthy sleep habits and seeking medical advice when sleep issues persist is crucial for maintaining overall well-being.

11.2 Strategies for Managing Fatigue and Daytime Sleepiness

Managing fatigue and daytime sleepiness requires a comprehensive approach that addresses both lifestyle modifications and potential underlying medical conditions. Here are some strategies to consider:

Prioritize Sleep: Aim for 7-9 hours of quality sleep each night. Establish a consistent sleep schedule by going to bed and waking up at the same times every day, even on weekends.

Create a Restful Sleep Environment: Make your bedroom conducive to sleep by keeping it cool, dark, and quiet. Invest in a comfortable mattress and pillows, and remove electronic devices that emit blue light.

Limit Screen Time: Avoid screens (phones, tablets, computers, TVs) at least an hour before bedtime, as the blue light emitted can interfere with the production of melatonin, a hormone that regulates sleep.

Mindful Eating: Avoid heavy meals close to bedtime, as digestion can disrupt sleep. Opt for light snacks if needed. Limit caffeine and alcohol intake, especially in the hours leading up to sleep.

Regular Exercise: Engaging in regular physical activity can improve sleep quality. Aim for at least 30 minutes of moderate exercise most days, but avoid intense workouts close to bedtime.

Stress Management: Practice relaxation techniques such as deep breathing, meditation, or yoga to help manage stress and improve sleep quality.

Napping Wisely: If you need to nap during the day, keep it short (20-30 minutes) and avoid napping too close to bedtime, as it can interfere with nighttime sleep.

Avoid Long Days: Try to maintain a balanced schedule that doesn't require excessively long workdays or late-night activities.

Cognitive Behavioral Therapy for Insomnia (CBT-I): This structured therapy helps identify and address negative thought patterns and behaviors that contribute to insomnia.

Consult a Healthcare Professional: If fatigue and daytime sleepiness persist despite lifestyle changes, consult a healthcare provider. Underlying medical conditions such as sleep apnea, restless legs syndrome, or insomnia might require specific treatment approaches.

Medication: In some cases, healthcare providers may prescribe medications to help manage sleep disorders. However, these should only be considered after other strategies have been explored and under the guidance of a medical professional.

Manage Shift Work: If you work irregular hours or night shifts, consult with your healthcare provider for strategies to help regulate your sleep-wake cycle.

Remember that individual responses to these strategies can vary, and it might take time to find the combination that works best for you. Consistency is key, and it's important to prioritize sleep as an essential component of overall health and well-being.

11.3 Creating a Sleep-Friendly Environment

Creating a sleep-friendly environment is crucial for ensuring restful and rejuvenating sleep. Here are some detailed steps to achieve that:

Optimal Lighting: Keep your bedroom's lighting soft and dim in the evening to signal to your body that it's time to wind down. Consider using blackout curtains to block out external light sources that might disturb your sleep.

Comfortable Bed: Invest in a good-quality mattress and pillows that provide adequate support and comfort. The right bedding can make a significant difference in the quality of your sleep.

Noise Control: Minimize disruptive noises by using earplugs, white noise machines, or calming sounds like rainfall or ocean waves. These can help drown out any disturbances and create a soothing auditory environment.

Temperature Regulation: Maintain a cool and comfortable room temperature. The ideal range is typically between 60 to 67 degrees Fahrenheit (15 to 19 degrees Celsius), as it promotes deeper sleep.

Limit Electronics: Keep electronic devices like smartphones, tablets, and computers out of the bedroom. The blue light emitted by screens can interfere with your body's production of melatonin, a hormone that regulates sleep.

Bedroom's Purpose: Reserve your bedroom primarily for sleep and intimacy. Avoid working, studying, or watching TV in bed, as these activities can disrupt your association of the bed with rest.

Declutter and Organize: A tidy and organized space can have a calming effect on the mind. Remove any clutter from your bedroom and create an environment that promotes relaxation.

Aromatherapy: Consider using calming scents like lavender or chamomile through essential oils for diffusers. These scents have been shown to have a positive impact on sleep quality.

Calm Color Palette: Opt for soothing and neutral colors on your bedroom walls and décor. Bright and stimulating colors might hinder relaxation.

Pre-Bedtime Routine: Establish a calming pre-sleep routine to signal to your body that it's time to wind down. This could include activities like reading, gentle stretching, or practicing relaxation techniques.

Limit Liquid Intake: Minimize drinking liquids close to bedtime to reduce the likelihood of waking up during the night for bathroom trips.

Avoid Heavy Meals and Stimulants: Refrain from heavy, spicy, or rich meals before bedtime. Additionally, limit caffeine and nicotine intake in the hours leading up to sleep.

Regular Sleep Schedule: Try to go to bed and wake up at the same time every day, even on weekends. Consistency helps regulate your body's internal clock.

Physical Activity: Engage in regular physical activity, but avoid intense workouts close to bedtime. Exercise earlier in the day can promote better sleep.

By incorporating these practices into your sleep routine and creating a sleep-conducive environment, you can significantly improve the quality of your sleep and wake up feeling more refreshed and energized.

Chapter 12

Long-Term Solutions for Snoring Prevention

Snoring is a common issue that can disrupt sleep and cause problems for both the person snoring and their sleeping partner. There are several long-term solutions that can help prevent or reduce snoring:

Lifestyle Changes: Making certain lifestyle changes can have a significant impact on snoring. Losing weight, especially if you're overweight, can reduce the amount of tissue in the throat that may be contributing to snoring. Avoiding alcohol and sedatives before bedtime can also help, as they relax the muscles in the throat and can lead to snoring.

Sleep Position: Sleeping on your back can cause the tongue and soft palate to collapse to the back of the throat, leading to snoring. Sleeping on your side can often alleviate this issue. Some people find it helpful to use pillows or devices that encourage side sleeping.

Nasal Congestion: If nasal congestion is contributing to your snoring, using saline nasal sprays or nasal strips to open up the nasal passages can be helpful. In some cases, medical treatment for chronic congestion, such as allergy medications or even surgery, might be necessary.

Oral Appliances: Dental devices that help position the jaw and tongue to keep the airway open during sleep can be effective for snoring caused by obstruction in the mouth and throat. These devices are usually custom-made by a dentist.

Continuous Positive Airway Pressure (CPAP) Therapy: CPAP machines are commonly used to treat sleep apnea, a condition often associated with snoring. They deliver a continuous stream of air pressure through a mask to keep the airway open.

Surgery: In cases where snoring is caused by structural issues, such as enlarged tonsils, a deviated septum, or excess tissue in the throat, surgical options may be considered. However, surgery is usually reserved for severe cases or when other treatments have failed.

Laser Therapy: Laser-assisted uvulopalatoplasty (LAUP) and other laser procedures can be used to tighten or remove excess tissue in the throat, reducing snoring. These procedures are often outpatient and minimally invasive.

Behavioral Therapy: For some individuals, snoring is linked to poor sleep habits or sleep disorders. Cognitive behavioral therapy for insomnia (CBT-I) can improve sleep quality and potentially reduce snoring.

Tongue Exercises: Strengthening the muscles of the tongue and throat through specific exercises can help prevent the collapse of these tissues during sleep.

Alternative Therapies: Some alternative therapies, such as playing certain musical instruments designed to strengthen throat muscles, have been proposed as potential solutions for snoring. However, their effectiveness is not widely established.

It's important to note that snoring can have various underlying causes, and what works for one person may not work for another. If snoring is persistent and disruptive, it's recommended to consult a medical professional or a sleep specialist for a thorough evaluation and personalized recommendations.

12.1 Maintaining Healthy Habits for Sustainable Results

Maintaining healthy habits for sustainable results is essential for long-term well-being. Consistency is key when it comes to healthy habits, whether it's related to exercise, nutrition, sleep, or stress management. Developing a routine that aligns with your goals and lifestyle is crucial.

Goal Setting: Start by setting clear, achievable goals. These could be related to weight loss, muscle gain, improved fitness, or stress reduction. Having specific goals helps you stay motivated and focused.

Gradual Changes: Rather than making drastic changes, introduce healthy habits gradually. This increases the likelihood of success and makes it easier to adapt to new routines.

Balanced Nutrition: Focus on a balanced diet that includes a variety of nutrients. Incorporate whole grains, lean proteins, fruits, vegetables, and healthy fats. Avoid extreme diets, as they are often unsustainable in the long run.

Regular Exercise: Find physical activities you enjoy and make them a regular part of your routine. Aim for a mix of cardiovascular, strength training, and flexibility exercises to improve overall fitness.

Consistent Sleep: Prioritize getting enough quality sleep. Create a sleep schedule that allows for 7-9 hours of rest each night. Adequate sleep supports recovery and overall health.

Stress Management: Practice stress-reduction techniques such as meditation, deep breathing, yoga, or spending time in nature. Chronic stress can undermine your efforts to maintain a healthy lifestyle.

Hydration: Drink plenty of water throughout the day. Staying hydrated supports bodily functions and can help control hunger.

Social Support: Surround yourself with a supportive network of friends, family, or workout buddies who encourage your healthy habits. Sharing your journey with others can provide motivation and accountability.

Tracking Progress: Keep track of your achievements and setbacks. Use a journal, app, or wearable device to monitor your exercise, nutrition, and other habits.

Flexibility and Adaptability: Life is full of changes and challenges. Be prepared to adapt your routine when necessary, while still staying committed to your overall goals.

Positive Mindset: Cultivate a positive attitude toward your health journey. Celebrate your successes and don't be too hard on yourself if you encounter setbacks.

Professional Guidance: If needed, seek guidance from healthcare professionals, nutritionists, or fitness trainers. Their expertise can help you make informed decisions and avoid common pitfalls.

Remember, maintaining healthy habits is a continuous process. It's about creating a lifestyle that supports your well-being, rather than focusing solely on short-term results. By prioritizing consistency, balance, and self-care, you can achieve sustainable and lasting improvements in your health and overall quality of life.

12.2 Monitoring and Managing Snoring Progress

Monitoring and managing snoring progress involves a comprehensive approach that combines lifestyle adjustments, medical interventions, and consistent monitoring. Here's an in-depth look at the strategies and steps involved:

Initial Assessment:
Start by understanding the severity of the snoring issue. Determine whether it's a simple snoring problem or if it's associated with a more serious condition like sleep apnea. Consult a medical professional for a thorough evaluation.

Lifestyle Modifications:

Weight Management: Excess weight, especially around the neck area, can contribute to snoring. Losing weight through a balanced diet and regular exercise can help reduce snoring.
Sleep Position: Sleeping on your back can cause the tongue and soft palate to collapse to the back of the throat, leading to snoring. Sleeping on your side can alleviate this issue.
Avoid Alcohol and Sedatives: These substances relax the muscles in the throat, increasing the likelihood of snoring. Avoid them, particularly close to bedtime.
Sleep Hygiene:

Consistent Sleep Schedule: Maintain a regular sleep schedule to regulate your body's internal clock.

Optimal Sleep Environment: Ensure your sleep environment is comfortable, quiet, and conducive to restful sleep.

Positional Therapy:

Anti-Snoring Pillows: These pillows are designed to encourage side-sleeping, helping to keep the airways open.

Wearable Devices: Some devices, like vests or belts, are designed to prevent you from sleeping on your back.

Medical Interventions:

Continuous Positive Airway Pressure (CPAP): If diagnosed with sleep apnea, a CPAP machine delivers a continuous stream of air to keep the airway open during sleep.

Mandibular Advancement Devices (MADs): These oral appliances reposition the lower jaw and tongue to prevent airway obstruction.

Surgery: In severe cases, surgical procedures like uvulopalatopharyngoplasty (UPPP) or genioglossus advancement (GA) may be considered to correct anatomical issues.

Regular Monitoring:

Sleep Diary: Maintain a sleep diary to track sleep patterns, snoring frequency, and any changes in lifestyle that might impact snoring.

Technology: Wearable devices or smartphone apps can monitor sleep quality and snoring events over time.

Follow-Up and Adjustments:

Regularly follow up with healthcare professionals to assess progress and make necessary adjustments to treatment plans.

If using devices like CPAP or MADs, ensure they are properly calibrated and fitting comfortably.

Long-Term Lifestyle Changes:

The strategies mentioned above should ideally become long-term habits to effectively manage snoring.

Continuously prioritize weight management, sleep positioning, and other lifestyle modifications to maintain progress.
Remember, the effectiveness of these approaches can vary based on individual factors. It's crucial to work closely with medical professionals to tailor a plan that suits your specific needs and addresses the underlying causes of snoring.

NOTES